Report on the Reporting Pathology Protocols for Colon and Rectum Cancers Project

Version Date: December 16, 2005

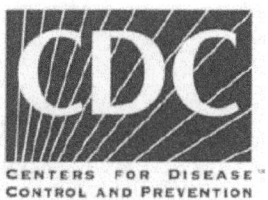

CDC

CENTERS FOR DISEASE
CONTROL AND PREVENTION

For more information, contact

National Program of Cancer Registries (NPCR)
National Center for Chronic Disease
Prevention and Health Promotion (NCCDPHP)
Centers for Disease Control and Prevention
4770 Buford Highway, MS K-53
Atlanta, Georgia 30341-3717
Phone: 770-488-4783
Fax: 770-488-4759
Web address: http://www.cdc.gov/cancer/npcr

<u>Table of Contents:</u>

Executive Summary

In 2001, the Centers for Disease Control and Prevention (CDC) National Program of Cancer Registries (NPCR) funded a pilot project involving two NPCR registries that partnered with two anatomical pathology (AP) laboratories. The intent of the pilot was to evaluate the use of structured data entry for cancer pathology reports for submission to cancer registries. The project included the California Cancer Registry collaborating with C/NET Solutions and the laboratory at the University of California at Irvine. Collaborating with the Ohio Cancer Incidence Surveillance System were the Rocky Mountain Cancer Data Systems (RMCDS) and the laboratory at University Hospitals of Cleveland. Additional participants included Cerner Dynamic Healthcare Technologies (DHT) and the Systematized Nomenclature of Medicine (SNOMED®) International, a division of the College of American Pathologists (CAP).

Pathology reports are typically in a text format with specific information contained in the narrative. To improve the quality and completeness of information in cancer pathology reports, CAP has developed 42 (as of 2004) site-specific cancer protocols and checklists for use by the pathology community. This project focused on implementing and improving the reporting of information from the SNOMED Clinical Terms® (SNOMED CT®) encoded CAP Colon and Rectum Cancer Checklists.

Software for the Reporting Pathology Protocols (RPP) project was developed to electronically capture the SNOMED CT encoded CAP Colorectal Cancer Checklists in participating AP laboratories. The project team established the structure of the project's Health Level 7 (HL7) message for both the core HL7 segments and the observation segments that corresponded to the data from the CAP Checklists. The RPP team maintained an open dialogue with the CAP Cancer Committee during the process of matching the CAP Checklist data to the corresponding HL7 observation segments. The data were entered by the laboratory team and then converted into the project standard HL7 Version 2.3.1 message. Next, data were transmitted to the participating cancer registry where the traditional narrative pathology report was evaluated and compared with the checklist data.

Using the SNOMED CT encoded CAP Cancer Checklists, either hard copy or electronically, is expected to provide significant advantages for the AP laboratory and cancer surveillance communities. Using the Checklists in a hospital pathology laboratory that is recognized by the Commission on Cancer (CoC) as an approved cancer program can help to ensure that Standard 4.6 is met: "The CoC requires that 90 percent of pathology reports that include a cancer diagnosis will contain the scientifically validated data elements outline on the surgical case summary checklist of the College of American Pathologists (CAP) publication, *Reporting on Cancer Specimens*." Receipt of the electronic version of the encoded checklists in cancer registries will reduce the tasks of coding and entering data from narrative text. Researchers who adopt the rapid case ascertainment systems of central cancer registries for special studies will find increased value in using these electronic checklists.

Electronic checklists make it possible to capture the intent of the pathologist at the point of diagnosis. Currently, cancer registrars often interpret text to derive the associated code. The electronic checklist allows data to be collected more accurately by standardizing the meaning of concepts and reporting data in a more timely manner.

Key Findings and Recommendations

In addition to CAP other organizations have developed cancer pathology checklists. The American College of Surgeons (ACoS) CoC requires cancer pathology reports to "contain the scientifically validated data elements outlined on the surgical case summary checklist" of the CAP Cancer Checklist publication. Other checklists or traditional text-based cancer pathology reports may also contain those data elements and are acceptable for meeting the CoC requirement. Cancer surveillance would substantially benefit from having a national standard for electronically transmitting pathology report checklist data to cancer registries.

1. **Recommendation:** CDC-NPCR encourages the ACoS CoC to revisit the requirements related to the CAP Cancer Checklists; to clarify those requirements, to explore mechanisms to promote electronic implementation of the CAP Cancer Checklists in hospital pathology laboratories, and transmission of those data to hospital cancer registries.

To demonstrate consistency with national HL7 conventions and standards, the RPP project used Logical Observation Identifiers Names and Codes (LOINC) as the question codes and SNOMED CT codes for the answers. "Question codes" generally refer to the code for a data item such as "Race". "Answer codes" refer to the data item's values such as the code for "White" or "Black" or "Chinese". At the start of this project LOINC codes did not exist for most of the CAP Checklist question (or data item) concepts. Participants identified the colon and rectum cancer CAP Checklist question concepts and presented them to the LOINC Clinical Committee. Codes for the colon and rectum cancer CAP Checklist questions were then issued and used within the project messages.

Currently, LOINC codes do not exist for many of the other (non-colorectal) cancer checklist question concepts. Examination of the SNOMED CT encoded checklists shows that SNOMED CT codes exist for the answer concepts as well as for the question concepts with the exception of some of the "other" text fields. This raises the issue, within the context of broader implementation of the CAP Cancer Checklists, of whether the LOINC question concepts are necessary for implementation of the HL7 message of the SNOMED CT encoded CAP Cancer Protocols and Checklists. This also raises a related question—which codes are AP laboratory information system (LIS) software developers and vendors currently using?

2. **Recommendation:** CDC-NPCR encourages national standard setters such as HL7, the Public Health Information Network (PHIN), and the North American Association of Central Cancer Registries (NAACCR) in collaboration with AP LIS vendors and developers; to investigate the HL7 message question/answer coding schema for synoptic cancer pathology reports, to describe current practices to establish national standards for the question codes, and for the answer codes.

One challenge facing the cancer surveillance community is identification of all cancers. Historically, a person trained in cancer identification visually scans each pathology and cytology report to identify a potential cancer. Implementation of the CAP Cancer Checklists can assist in the process of cancer identification however, not all cancers will be identified through this mechanism. For example, in situ cancers of the colon and rectum are not included in the CAP Cancer Checklists. Cancer registries collecting the SNOMED CT encoded CAP Cancer Checklist data will need to establish additional case-finding mechanisms to search for and identify cancers from pathology reports using the traditional narrative-text format.

3. **Recommendation:** CDC-NPCR encourages the CAP Cancer Committee to investigate systems within AP laboratories to assist with cancer registration case identification, especially for those reportable cancers currently without a CAP Cancer Checklist. One conceivable solution is to add the following question within the AP laboratory systems for the pathologist: "Should this report be reviewed by the cancer registry?"

Most AP laboratories contract with AP LIS vendors for pathology report-processing software. AP LIS vendors charge AP laboratories a licensing fee for the use of their software as well as additional fees for modules associated with the CAP Cancer Checklists. As demand for these products with the CAP Cancer Checklist capability increases and more vendors enter the marketplace, the vendor charges to AP laboratories should decrease.

4. **Recommendation:** CDC-NPCR encourages the CAP Cancer Committee and SNOMED International to promote the value of the SNOMED CT encoded CAP Cancer Protocols within the AP community.

5. **Recommendation:** CDC-NPCR encourages the national cancer surveillance and AP laboratory community to investigate alternative funding mechanisms for the SNOMED CT encoding costs associated with the CAP Checklists.

Some data items from the CAP Checklist are directly mappable into the cancer registry database. Others are not. For example, the CAP Checklist "Histologic Type" can be mapped to NAACCR data item "Histologic Type ICD-O-3," whereas the CAP Checklist "Additional Pathologic Findings" is not directly related to a particular NAACCR data item. From the cancer surveillance perspective, how should those data items not mappable to the cancer registry database be handled? How should the data from the CAP Cancer Checklists be incorporated into the cancer registry software systems?

6. **Recommendation:** CDC-NPCR recommends that NAACCR examine the usefulness of the CAP Cancer Checklist data items, identify those not needed from the cancer registry systems, and map the CAP Checklist data items designated as appropriate to the corresponding NAACCR data item.

7. **Recommendation:** CDC-NPCR recommends that cancer registry software vendors and developers, in collaboration with cancer registry staff, design and develop systems to accept electronic cancer pathology report data from AP laboratories in both traditional text format and in CAP Cancer Checklist format.

8. **Recommendation:** CDC-NPCR recommends that NPCR registries implement systems to collect electronic cancer pathology report data in both traditional text format and in CAP Cancer Checklist format.

The CAP Cancer Checklist data items could also form the basis for an anatomical pathology laboratory database. Such a database could be linked to the cancer registry database producing a more robust research tool.

9. **Recommendation:** CDC-NPCR recommends that AP LIS developers and vendors design mechanisms to maintain the CAP Cancer Checklist data items in an AP laboratory database.

The intent of the CAP Cancer Checklists was to provide pathologists with a format to ensure the complete capture of essential elements and to increase accuracy. The checklists were never intended to prohibit the inclusion of descriptive text in the cancer pathology report. Clinical history is an example of useful cancer surveillance information that is typically included in narrative text and not contained in the checklists. Allowing text, in addition to the checklist data items, could encourage pathologists to use the associated checklist software. Discussions with AP LIS vendors indicate that this is the current strategy for product design.

10. **Recommendation:** CDC-NPCR recommends that AP LIS developers and vendors include text fields with the cancer checklist data items.

Obtaining consensus on the location of information from the CAP Cancer Checklists in the HL7 observation segment, as well as the location of other header, patient, and physician identification information in the appropriate HL7 segments, was a time-consuming challenge. During the course of this project, NAACCR initiated a project to develop an HL7 message standard for the traditional narrative style pathology reports. In April 2005, NAACCR released a draft document entitled "Implementation Guide for Transmission of Laboratory Based Reports to Cancer Registries using Version 2.3.1 of the HL7 Standards Protocol." The document addresses many of the same issues identified during this project.

11. **Recommendation:** CDC-NPCR recommends that NAACCR expand the pathology laboratory electronic reporting implementation guide to include guidance on the structure of CAP Cancer Checklist data message.

In the colon and rectum CAP Cancer Checklists, there was a loss of histology specificity, primarily those related to adenocarcinoma arising in an adenoma. The CAP colorectal cancer checklist limits the number of histologies to a choice of seven, with an option to insert text. There are many possible histologies for colorectal cancers. The idea behind limited lists is to offer the most common choices and for pathologists to chose the "Other (specify)" option for less common histologies. In general, use of the "Other (specify)" concepts tends to result in underreporting.

12. **Recommendation:** CDC-NPCR recommends that AP LIS developers and vendors designing and developing electronic versions of the CAP Cancer Checklists use drop-down lists including all the site-specific histologies in addition to the main histology codes. These tables are available at the National Cancer Institute Surveillance Epidemiology and End Results (NCI SEER) web site: http://seer.cancer.gov/icd-o-3/.

The CAP Checklists contain the appropriate Tumor - Node - Metastasis (TNM) codes for each checklist site. However, the Collaborative Staging (CS) data items were not incorporated into the CAP Cancer Checklists.

13. **Recommendation:** CDC-NPCR recommends that future pilot projects designed to implement the CAP Cancer Checklists map the CAP Cancer Checklist data items to the CS data items, to assess the completeness of the CAP Cancer Checklists for CS. Findings should be presented to the CAP Cancer Committee with a request to include the relevant data items in future iterations of the CAP Cancer Checklists.

Although regional lymph node involvement is included in the CAP Colon and Rectum cancer checklist, the location of the regional lymph node chain is not included. What is the value of the specific regional lymph node chain for cancer surveillance? Why is this information included in the Surveillance Epidemiology and End Results (SEER) Extent of Disease (EOD) and CS Lymph Node data items but not in the CAP colon and rectum cancer checklist? In short, how significant is this loss of specificity?

14. **Recommendation:** CDC-NPCR recommends that the American Joint Committee on Cancer (AJCC) and the CAP Cancer Committee explore the value of the name of the specific regional lymph node chain for cancer surveillance and clinical purposes and recommend adjustments to the CS schema and the CAP Cancer Checklists. Although this recommendation focuses on the CAP Colon and Rectum Cancer Checklists, it may also be an issue with CAP Cancer Checklists for other sites.

Two of the choices in the CAP Colon and Rectum Cancer Checklist under Histologic Type include Mucinous adenocarcinoma and Signet-ring cell carcinoma with some qualifiers— "Mucinous adenocarcinoma (greater than 50% mucinous)" and "Signet-ring cell carcinoma (greater than 50% signet-ring cells)." The corresponding guidance for cancer registrars is not as specific as the CAP Checklist's "50%" criteria. There may be a discrepancy between the coding rules used by pathologists in the CAP Checklist and those used by cancer registrars.

15. **Recommendation:** CDC-NPCR recommends that the AJCC, CAP Cancer Committee, and SEER examine histology coding rules in greater detail and ensure that coding rules are consistent among pathologists and cancer registrars. Although this recommendation focuses on the CAP Colon and Rectum Cancer Checklists, it may also be an issue with CAP Cancer Checklists for other sites.

The CAP Checklists contain some codes in addition to the standard TNM codes: pT3a/b and pT3c/d. These codes are not part of the AJCC TNM Manual, but they are part of *TNM*

Supplement. A Commentary on Uniform Use (2nd edition) and are included in the chapter "Optional Proposals for Testing New Telescopic Ramifications of TNM."

16. **Recommendation:** CDC-NPCR recommends that the cancer registry software developers and vendors be aware of the TNM codes included in *TNM Supplement, A Commentary on Uniform Use* and convert those codes to the most appropriate TNM code (i.e., pT3). Although this recommendation focuses on the CAP Colon and Rectum Cancer Checklists, it may also be an issue with CAP Cancer Checklists for other sites.

A need was identified for the cancer registry software developers to be able to receive and process the checklists. As part of this process, the cancer registry software developers must know which checklist is being received. At the request of the RPP team, SNOMED provided a "Checklist Identifier" concept code for each checklist. This concept better enables software developers to receive electronic versions of this information to incorporate the data into the cancer registry software as well as other systems. This Checklist Identifier concept has now been added to all the SNOMED CT encoded CAP Checklists.

Conclusions

This project required a considerable amount of time to allow for a process of acculturation among team members. Because of the nature of the project, expertise was drawn from people with several highly specialized fields: cancer registration, pathology, AP laboratory management, laboratory information systems, the CAP Cancer Protocols and Checklists, and the SNOMED CT terminology. The team members were accustomed to specialized language and unique perspectives. It took considerable time to develop a common language to bridge disciplines and to widen viewpoints to establish the kind of communication needed to move RPP ahead. This was particularly true regarding the fine points of messaging and coding and finding common ground between the needs of pathologists and the needs of cancer registrars. The CAP Checklists and the HL7 message standards were new tools for most of the team members, which added to the learning curve. All these aspects of project development were necessary and time-consuming but essential to the success of the effort. In summary, the RPP team had to develop the ability to think in common terms from a common perspective using new tools before it could begin to move toward project goals.

RPP Team Members

Mary Abbuhl, University Hospitals of Cleveland, Department of Pathology
Linda Coles, Cerner-DHT Corporation
Michele Connors, Cerner-DHT Corporation
Kathleen Davidson-Allen, California Cancer Registry
Ken Gerlach, CDC-National Program of Cancer Registries
Barry Gordon, C/NET Solutions
Georgette Haydu, Ohio Cancer Incidence Surveillance System
Zeke Holland, Cerner-DHT Corporation
Mark Jordan, Cerner-DHT Corporation
Mary Kennedy, SNOMED International

John Kilbourne, SNOMED International
Fritz Lin, University of California at Irvine, Department of Pathology
Pat Patterson, University Hospitals of Cleveland, Department of Pathology
Bette Smith, Ohio Cancer Incidence Surveillance System
Corey Smith, SNOMED International
Dieter Thum, Cerner-DHT Corporations
Monique van Berkum, SNOMED International
Joseph Willis, University Hospitals of Cleveland Pathology and Case Western Reserve University

Overview

National Program of Cancer Registries and National Standards

The National Program of Cancer Registries (NPCR) was authorized by the Cancer Registries Amendment Act, Public Law (PL) 102-515, and is administered by CDC-NPCR's Division of Cancer Prevention and Control. The funds were awarded to support states in their efforts to enhance state cancer registries or to plan and implement cancer registries if they did not exist. NPCR currently supports population-based cancer registries in 45 states, the District of Columbia, and 3 U.S. territories. Since the inception of NPCR, participating central cancer registries and affiliated hospitals are required to report and use a standard nationally defined set of specific data items and codes.

These national data item definitions and associated format standards have been defined by the North American Association of Central Cancer Registries (NAACCR), an association of state cancer registries and national cancer registry organizations including, among others, CDC-NPCR; the National Cancer Institute (NCI) Surveillance, Epidemiology, and End Results (SEER) program; Statistics Canada; and the American College of Surgeons (ACoS) Commission on Cancer (CoC). The NAACCR Data Standards and Data Dictionary are located on the NAACCR web site at http://www.naaccr.org/.

Cancer Registration and the Importance of Pathology Reporting

Population-based cancer registration is a key tool for cancer control. PL 102-515 notes, "cancer control programs and existing statewide population-based cancer registries have identified cancer incidence and cancer mortality rates that indicate the burden of cancer for Americans is substantial and varies widely by geographic location and by ethnicity." This law requires participating states to provide authorization under state law for the statewide cancer registry to ensure the complete reporting of cancer cases to the statewide cancer registry by physicians, surgeons, and all other health care practitioners diagnosing or providing treatment for cancer patients.

Reporting cancer data starts with the date of diagnosis (or a little earlier) and ends when treatment is complete. Typically, staff in hospital cancer registries review the data in the hospital medical record, record the pertinent text information, code the reportable data items, assess the quality of the data item codes, and submit the report to the central cancer registry or population-based cancer registry. In reporting facilities without cancer registries, individuals are required to complete a similar process. There are several sources for identifying cancers, including the hospitals' disease index (list of diseases by ICD-9-CM codes), radiation therapy logs, billing logs, and pathology laboratory reports (including cytology and hematology). Of these sources, the primary or key source is the anatomical pathology laboratory.

In the United States, more than 90% of all cancers are microscopically confirmed. "At any time during the patient's medical history there was microscopic confirmation of the morphology of this cancer" (*The SEER Program Code Manual*, 3rd edition, 1/98). Microscopically confirmed includes diagnoses based on tissue specimens from biopsy, frozen section, surgery, autopsy, dilation and curettage; peripheral blood smears; bone marrow specimens; and cytologic diagnoses including smears from sputum, bronchial brushings, bronchial washings, tracheal washings, breast secretions, spinal fluid, peritoneal fluid, pleural fluid, and urine. Pathology laboratories (including cytology and hematology) are critically important for complete and timely identification of cancer cases and have the potential to serve as the basis for rapid ascertainment of cancer cases.

CAP Cancer Protocols and Checklists

In April 1999, CAP, with the leadership of the CAP Cancer Committee, published[1] "aid the surgical pathologist with completeness, accuracy, and uniformity in the reporting of malignant tumor specimens and with quality assurance issues related to such specimens. They may be used as a framework for full narrative reporting, alternative reporting formats, or clinical research protocols. The accompanying surgical pathology case summaries (checklists) represent synoptic forms of the information contained in each protocol, and like the protocols themselves, are tailored to individual specimen types (e.g., cytology, diagnostic biopsy, excisional biopsy or resection)." These protocols and the associated checklists are intended to be guidelines for pathologists. The protocols at that time (1999) included 22 site-specific checklists. At the time of this project (2004), there were 42 such site-specific checklists with more under development. The checklists distinguish between data items required by CAP (essential data elements) and those that are optional. These checklists are available for individual use by pathologists at the web site http://www.cap.org/apps/docs/cancer_protocols/protocols_index.html. Using the checklists for commercial purposes requires a license. Information about the copyrights of these products from CAP is included in the introduction to Appendix A. The web site referenced above contains the Full Protocols" as well as the "Checklists". The Full Protocols contain the Checklists, as well as background documentation, explanatory notes, and references. The Colon and Rectum Cancer Protocol contains three separate checklists: Colon and Rectum: Polypectomy, Rectum: Local Excision (Transanal Disk Excision), and Colon and Rectum: Resection.

Typically, anatomical pathology reports are in free-form narrative text. For example, a final diagnosis may read as follows: "Colon, right, segmental resection to include appendix and ileum: Mucinous adenocarcinoma invading through the bowel wall into the pericolonic adipose tissue. Margins are free of tumor. Benign appendix. All of twenty-two lymph nodes are free of tumor.

---

[1] *Reporting on Cancer Specimens Protocols and Case Summaries.* The protocols p. 7

TNM stage pT3 pN0 pMX." A cancer registry professional, who determines the reportability of the report and codes the concepts as needed, usually processes this information. Text-searching software is available to identify reportable tumors and code-specific concepts, but it tends to be expensive.

Below is an example of a section from the colon-rectum checklist. The complete checklist is included in the appendices.

Colon and Rectum

Protocol applies to all invasive carcinomas of the colon and rectum. Carcinoid tumors, lymphomas, sarcomas, and tumors of the vermiform appendix are excluded.

Protocol revision date: January 2004
Based on AJCC/UICC TNM, 6th edition

Colon and Rectum: Polypectomy

Patient name:
Surgical pathology number:

Note: Check 1 response unless otherwise indicated.

Macroscopic

Tumor Site

___ Cecum
___ Right (ascending) colon
___ Hepatic flexure
___ Transverse colon
___ Splenic flexure
___ Left (descending) colon
___ Sigmoid colon
___ Rectum
___ Not specified

Polyp Size

Greatest dimension: ___ cm
*Additional dimensions: ___ x ___ cm
___ Cannot be determined (see Comment)

ACoS CoC Standards

ACoS CoC accredits more than 1,400 cancer treatment centers in the United States. As part of that accreditation process, treatment centers are required to meet Cancer Program Standards. The CoC "sets standards for quality multidisciplinary cancer care delivered primarily in hospital settings; surveys facilities to assess compliance with those standards; collects standardized and quality data from approved facilities to measure treatment patterns and outcomes; and uses the data to evaluate hospital provider performance and develop effective educational interventions to improve cancer care outcomes at the national and local levels[2]"

Starting with cancers diagnosed on or after January 1, 2004, pathologists in CoC accredited treatment centers are required to incorporate the CAP cancer protocol and checklist essential data elements. Specifically, Standard 4.6 notes, "The CoC requires that 90 percent of pathology reports that include a cancer diagnosis will contain the scientifically validated data elements outlined on the surgical case summary checklist of the College of American Pathologists (CAP) publication, reporting on Cancer Specimens.[3]" At the May 2004 CoC meeting, additional clarification was added, "inspections are limited to cancer-directed surgical resection specimens only. Cytologic specimens, diagnostic biopsies, and palliative resection specimens are excluded.[4]"

Systematized Nomenclature of Medicine Clinical Terms (SNOMED CT)

SNOMED CT is a scientifically validated clinical health care terminology. The SNOMED CT ore terminology provides a common language that enables a consistent way of capturing, sharing, and aggregating health data. Among the applications for SNOMED CT are electronic medical records, clinical decision support, medical research studies, clinical trials, computerized physician order entry, disease surveillance, image indexing, and consumer health information services.

SNOMED International, a division of CAP maintains the SNOMED CT technical design, the core content architecture, and the SNOMED CT core content. The SNOMED CT core terminology contains more than 361,800 health care concepts with unique meanings and formal logic-based definitions organized into hierarchies. As of January 2004, the fully populated table with unique descriptions for each concept contained more than 975,000 descriptions. Approximately 1.47 million semantic relationships exist to enable reliability and consistency of data retrieval.

SNOMED CT is comprehensive, but it can map to other medical terminologies and classification systems, which avoids duplicate data capture, while facilitating enhanced health reporting, billing, and statistical analysis. SNOMED CT also provides a framework to manage language dialects, clinically relevant subsets, qualifiers, and extensions as well as concepts and terms unique to particular organizations or localities. SNOMED CT combines the content and structure of the SNOMED Reference Terminology (SNOMED RT) with the United Kingdom's Clinical Terms Version 3 (formerly known as the Read Codes).

In 2003, CAP signed a 5-year sole source contract with the National Library of Medicine (NLM) to license English and Spanish language editions of SNOMED CT. NLM is part of the National Institutes of Health within the U.S. Department of Health and Human Services. Since the first

---

[2] Commission on Cancer, *Cancer Program Standards 2004*, p. 1
[3] Commission on Cancer, *Cancer Program Standards 2004*, p. 38
[4] *CAP Today*, June 2004, Vol. 18, No. 6, p. 58

quarter of 2004, free-of-charge access to SNOMED CT core content and all version updates for covered entities has been available through NLM's Unified Medical Language System Metathesaurus (a knowledge source containing biomedical concepts and terms from many controlled vocabularies and classifications). Under the agreement, SNOMED CT will continue to be available directly from SNOMED International in the original SNOMED CT structure.

On December 7, 1999, CAP was approved as an American National Standards Institute (ANSI) accredited Standards Developer Organization. The CAP activity relating to clinical terminology, through SNOMED International, focuses on standardizing terminology across clinical specialties and sites of care. These standards are developed in response to the increasing need to document care in a computer-readable format, to reliably and reproducibly retrieve and aggregate patient level and population-based data, and to transmit data in electronic format.

On September 30, 2003, CAP received ANSI approval for the Healthcare Terminology Structure Standard. This standard specifies a standard file structure for use in distributing health care terminology.

As a continuation of its Health Insurance and Accountability Act of 1996 mandate, the National Committee on Vital and Health Statistics (NCVHS) assessed clinical terminology standards for the patient medical record initiative (PMRI). In 2003, the NCVHS Subcommittee on Standards and Security completed a detailed evaluation of 38 health care terminologies and classification systems to support the electronic medical record. Ten terminologies met all the essential criteria defined according to sound medical informatics practices. SNOMED CT was rated highest of the terminologies evaluated.

On November 12, 2003, an advisory panel of the Department of Health and Human Services recommended SNOMED CT as part of a core set of PMRI terminology. In the letter about PMRI terminology, the NCVHS said, "The breadth of content, sound terminology model and widely recognized value of SNOMED CT qualify it as a general-purpose terminology for the exchange, aggregation, and analysis of patient medical information. The broad scope of SNOMED CT itself and the inclusion within it of concepts from other important health care terminologies (including the following terminologies developed to support nursing practice: HHCC, NANDA, NOC, NIC, Omaha System, and PNS) allow SNOMED CT to encompass much of the patient medical record information domain."

On January 29, 2004, the Consolidated Health Informatics Initiative recommended and endorsed SNOMED CT as the terminology of choice for the domains of anatomy, nursing, diagnosis and problems, and non-laboratory interventions and procedures.

CAP is a member of HL7 and actively contributes to the coordination of HL7 messaging standards and SNOMED CT content. SNOMED CT is a registered standard with the HL7 Vocabulary Technical Committee for use in HL7 messages.

SNOMED CT Encoded Checklists

CAP offers the SNOMED CT encoded CAP Cancer Checklists to assist surgical pathologists in reporting the most common forms of adult cancer and for effectively delivering the information necessary to provide quality patient care. The CAP Cancer Checklists are synoptic or structured reports designed to ensure that findings are standardized to provide complete and consistent information to clinicians. SNOMED International has enhanced the CAP checklists by encoding them on an item-by-item basis with SNOMED CT. The SNOMED CT encoded Cancer Checklists are an electronic enrichment of the CAP Cancer Checklists.

Below is an example of a section from the 2004 SNOMED CT encoded colon-rectum checklist. The entire colon and rectum checklist is included in Appendix A. The non-italicized text represents literal text from the CAP Cancer Checklist while the italicized text represents the SNOMED CT encoded identifiers and fully specified names for those items.

COLON AND RECTUM: Resection *[P1-573F9, 107944001] Large intestine excision (procedure)*

MACROSCOPIC *[F-048D6, 395526000] Macroscopic specimen observable (observable entity)*

SPECIMEN TYPE *[R-00254, 371439000] Specimen type (observable entity)*
___ Right hemicolectomy *[G-8371, 122648004] Specimen from colon obtained by right hemicolectomy (specimen)*
    *Length: ___ cm *[R-00408, 384606002] Length of specimen (observable entity)*
___ Transverse colectomy *[G-8372, 122649007] Specimen from colon obtained by transverse colectomy (specimen)*
    *Length: ___ cm *[R-00408, 384606002] Length of specimen (observable entity)*
___ Left hemicolectomy *[G-8373, 122650007] Specimen from colon obtained by left hemicolectomy (specimen)*
    *Length: ___ cm *[R-00408, 384606002] Length of specimen (observable entity)*
___ Sigmoidectomy *[G-8374, 122651006] Specimen from colon obtained by sigmoidectomy (specimen)*
    *Length: ___ cm *[R-00408, 384606002] Length of specimen (observable entity)*
___ Rectal/rectosigmoid colon (low anterior resection) *[G-8375, 122652004] Specimen from colon obtained by rectal/rectosigmoid (low anterior) resection (specimen)*
    *Length: ___ cm *[R-00408, 384606002] Length of specimen (observable entity)*
___ Total abdominal colectomy *[G-8369, 122647009] Specimen from large intestine obtained by total abdominal colectomy (specimen)*
    *Length: ___ cm *[R-00408, 384606002] Length of specimen (observable entity)*
___ Abdominoperineal resection *[G-8368, 122646000] Specimen from large intestine obtained by abdominoperineal resection (specimen)*
    *Length: ___ cm *[R-00408, 384606002] Length of specimen (observable entity)*
___ Other (specify): ___ *not coded*
    *Length: ___ cm *[R-00408, 384606002] Length of specimen (observable entity)*
___ Not specified *[G-8365, 122643008] Tissue specimen from large intestine (specimen)*

Project Logistics

In October 2001 in response to Program Announcement (PA) 01102, Cancer Surveillance Research and Data Enhancement and Utilization—Notice of Funds, CDC-National Program of Cancer Registries (NPCR) awarded funds to the California Department of Health Services in Collaboration with the Public Health Institute and the Ohio Department of Health to participate in a 3-year pilot project entitled "Reporting Pathology Protocols for Colon and Rectum Cancers." PA 01102 applicants were limited to NPCR registries that could demonstrate through a letter of support at least one effective partnership with a laboratory or laboratory vendor providing pathologic diagnostic services in a National Cancer Institute (NCI) designated comprehensive cancer or clinical cancer center facility in their state.

The purpose of this project was to use an electronic data entry program or input screen of the College of American Pathologists (CAP) colon and rectum cancer protocol checklists for use by pathologists in a participating hospital anatomical pathology laboratory, to convert those data into a message consistent with national data standards, and to transmit the data to the participating cancer registry.

The activities of the participants per PA 01102 are noted below.

1. Develop, in collaboration with other successful recipients, strategies to implement the CAP reporting protocols for cancers of the colon and rectum.
2. Develop electronic reporting capacities to relate data from the protocols to an appropriate cancer registry.
3. Implement CAP reporting protocols for cancers of the colon and rectum.
4. Participate with other successful applicants and key groups to share expertise and experiences.
5. Provide written feedback and recommendations about the protocols to improve the protocols for cancers of the colon and rectum that will meet the needs of pathologists and cancer registries.

The following diagram describes the generic project workflow.

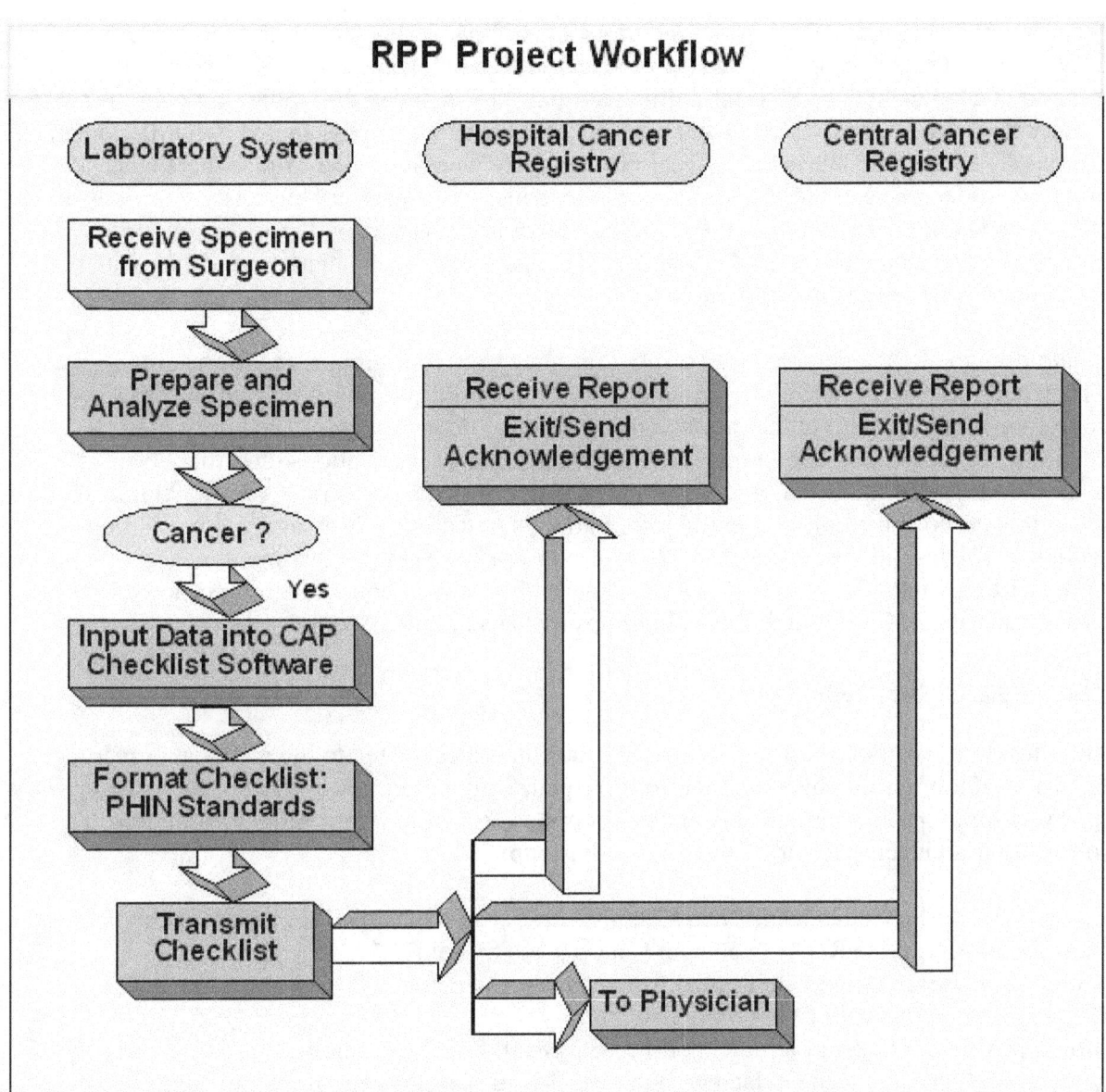

California and Ohio offered different mechanisms to accomplish the project's mission. These models or workflows are noted in the sections California Implementation Workflow and Ohio Implementation Workflow.

The earlier reference to a "message consistent with national data standards" refers to a number of endeavors including the CDC-NPCR Public Health Information Network (PHIN) standards. CDC-NPCR, in conjunction with national partners, has identified standards as described in the PHIN. PHIN is a CDC-NPCR-led effort to improve public health communications by using and promoting health data and technology standards. The intent is to provide and exchange timely information at all levels of public health. Additional information about PHIN can be obtained at the following web site: http://www.cdc.gov/phin/.

To accomplish the project's mission, the project participants and staff from SNOMED International, the reporting pathology protocols (RPP) team, met on a regular basis to discuss issues and challenges. The SNOMED International staff included those working with the CAP Cancer Committee on the CAP cancer protocol checklists and the associated SNOMED Clinical Terms (CT) encoding. During the 3-year project, there were four face-to-face meetings and monthly conference call meetings. One of the meetings took place at University Hospitals of Cleveland and included a tour of the pathology laboratory, starting with the macroscopic description of specimens by residents and surgical pathology technicians and ending with the dictation of final reports by the pathologists.

In addition, the RPP team formed two sub-committees or work groups: the Messaging Work Group and the Assessment Work Group. The task of the Messaging Work Group was to obtain consensus on the content of the message using national data standards. The group used HL7 version 2.3.1 as the message format with LOINC (Logical Observations Identifiers Names and Codes) codes as the questions and SNOMED CT codes as the answers. (Additional information about this group and message specific information is noted in the Messaging Work Group section.) The task of the Assessment Work Group was to develop assessment measures for each of the participating NPCR registries. (Additional information about this group is noted in the Assessment Work Group section.) Both groups met as needed.

Messaging Work Group

The Messaging Work Group was formed to focus on issues related to the message or record format used to transmit checklist data from the pathology laboratory to the cancer registry. The goal was for all project participants to use a common format to transmit the information. The following individuals participated in this work group:

Linda Coles, Zeke Holland, and Dieter Thum with Cerner Dynamic Healthcare Technologies
Larry Derrick with the Rocky Mountain Cancer Data System
Kathleen Davidson-Allen with the California Cancer Registry
Barry Gordon with C/NET Corporation
Monique Van Berkum and John Kilbourne with SNOMED International
Warren Williams and Ken Gerlach with the CDC-National Program of Cancer Registries

Relying on the PHIN standards as an overarching guide, the work group agreed to use Health Level 7 (HL7) Version 2.3.1 as the message format with Logical Observation Identifier Names and Codes (LOINC) codes as the questions and Systematized Nomenclature of Medicine Clinical Terms (SNOMED CT) codes as the answers. The first step in the process was to review the College of American Pathologists (CAP) Cancer Checklists to identify those concepts on the checklist without an associated LOINC question code. These concepts were presented to the Clinical LOINC Committee and codes were created for these concepts and incorporated into the project messaging tables.

The CAP Colon and Rectum Cancer checklists were also reviewed. The checklists were originally designed as paper forms and not as software. The checklist paper form was able to capture (through indentation) whether more than one item could be checked because at times a subtype of a checklist item could also be chosen.

The checklists, in general, allow for only one response per section unless the option to choose more than one answer for a section is indicated (e.g., a "check all that apply" option is indicated for the "Venous (Large Vessel) Invasion (V)" section of the checklist shown below).

VENOUS (LARGE VESSEL) INVASION (V) (check all that apply)
___ Absent
___ Present
  *___ Intramural
  *___ Extramural
___ Indeterminate

Sometimes, the formatting of the checklist added context to the "check all that apply" option. For the example above, the only reason for the option "check all that apply" is to allow for an optional subtype of "Present" (either "Intramural" or "Extramural") to be selected as well. There is an "if-then" type of structure implied by the indentation of "Intramural" and "Extramural" with respect to "Present". If you chose "Present" then you have the option of choosing one of its subtype choices. "Check all that apply" is not intended to allow the user to select more than one of the three main choices. Capturing this type of formatting context of the paper checklist was a software design challenge.

Another challenging situation occurs with a section that has optional sub-questions allowing for more detail. For some of these sub-questions, it was unclear whether they were required or optional. For the "Margins" example shown below, the last two questions "Distance of invasive carcinoma from closest margin: ___ mm OR ___ cm" and "Specify margin: ____" can be answered only if all the margin choices offered were uninvolved by tumor. Yet, the last two questions are not asterisked so they appear to be mandatory. The implied context is that they are mandatory but only if all of the listed margins were uninvolved by tumor.

MARGINS (check all that apply)

Proximal Margin
___Cannot be assessed
___ Uninvolved by invasive carcinoma
___ Involved by invasive carcinoma
___ Carcinoma in situ/adenoma absent at proximal margin
___ Carcinoma in situ/adenoma present at proximal margin

Distal Margin
___Cannot be assessed
___ Uninvolved by invasive carcinoma
___ Involved by invasive carcinoma
___ Carcinoma in situ/adenoma absent at distal margin
___ Carcinoma in situ/adenoma present at distal margin

Circumferential (Radial) Margin
___ Not applicable
___ Cannot be assessed
___ Uninvolved by invasive carcinoma
___ Involved by invasive carcinoma (tumor present 0–1 mm from circumferential radial margin)

*Mesenteric Margin
*___ Cannot be assessed
*___ Uninvolved by invasive carcinoma
*___ Involved by invasive carcinoma

Distance of invasive carcinoma from closest margin: ___ mm OR ___ cm
Specify margin: ____

The information inherent in the paper form had to be translated into appropriate business rules and the associated software design. Interaction with the CAP Cancer Committee resulted in clarification of these issues in some cases and adjustments to future versions of the checklists in other cases. For the example given above, in a later version of the checklist, the following change was made for clarification.

"Distance of invasive carcinoma from closest margin: ___ mm OR ___ cm
Specify margin: ____ "

was changed to:

"If all margins uninvolved by invasive carcinoma:
Distance of invasive carcinoma from closest margin: ___ mm OR ___ cm
Specify margin: _____."

The meetings of the Messaging Work Group revolved around reaching consensus on two messaging tables: the OBX table and the Fields table. The OBX (HL7 OBX = observation) table reflects the work to map the concepts or data items on the CAP Colon and Rectum Checklists into specific HL7 message segments. This table is located in Appendix D; a portion of that table is noted below.

RPP Item #	Proposed Item Name for Messaging	CAP Checklist Item Name	LOINC code	Data type*	SNOMED code
4	Tumor Site	Tumor Site	33725-3	CE	371480007
11	Histologic Type	Histologic Type	31205-8	CWE	371441004

13	Histologic Grade (hi/low)	Histologic Grade	33732-9	CWE	371469007

The RPP Fields table reflects the work to incorporate other HL7 segments into the standard message or record format. These other segments included the following: message header (MSH), patient identification (PID), patient visit (PV1), order common information (ORC), observation request (OBR), and additional observation (OBX). This table is located in Appendix C; a portion of the table is noted below.

HL7 ID Number	HL7 Name	HL7 Req	RPP Req	Ohio Uses	Calif. Uses	Contents, Format, or Example	Data Type
MSH:01	Field Separator	R	R	R	R	|	ST
MSH:02	Encoding Characters	R	R	R	R	"^~&"	ST
MSH:03	Sending Application	R	R	R	R	"CNETRPP" or "CoPathPlus"	HD
MSH:04	Sending Facility	R	R	R	R	Path Facility ID # (CLIA #) Name^Code^CLIA	HD
MSH:05	Receiving Application	O	O	Y	Y	e.g., "Cancer Registry Application"	HD
MSH:06	Receiving Facility	O	O	Y	Y	"UCI" or "State Cancer Registry"	HD
MSH:07	Date/Time of Message	R	R	R	R	YYYYMMDDHHMMSS	TS

During the Messaging Work Group meetings, a number of messaging issues and questions were discussed. The questions, the associated discussion, and the decision are included in the appendices. The questions are grouped into three general headings: HL7 Message, Unresolved, and Checklist. See Appendix F.

One challenge was to incorporate the updates made to the CAP cancer checklists by the CAP Cancer Committee. The CAP Cancer Checklists are updated once a year, in January, whereas SNOMED CT is released twice a year, in January and July. Therefore, a limited number of the SNOMED CT codes could change in the July and January release due to changes in the terminology, whereas the CAP un-encoded Checklists would only potentially change on a yearly basis. This created a number of versioning issues for the message, which to date are not resolved.

In addition, other checklist changes were initiated at the request of the RPP project. For example, as the project evolved it became apparent that a unique checklist identifier was needed for each of the checklists. Within the Colon and Rectum Checklist, for example, there are actually three distinct checklists: Colon and Rectum: Polypectomy, Rectum: Local Excision (Transanal Disk

Excision), Colon and Rectum: Resection. SNOMED CT created individual codes to identify each CAP Checklist and added these in the January 2004 version of the SNOMED CT encoded CAP Checklists. As new question concepts were added to the checklist, the project was challenged to obtain and incorporate LOINC question codes for the new concepts.

After agreement on the content of the two tables, the laboratory software developers create alpha test messages to exchange with each other to ensure that the messages followed the agreed upon specifications. These alpha test messages (de-identified) are included in Appendix E.

Assessment Work Group

The Assessment Work Group was formed to focus on issues related to assessment or evaluation of the project. The main overarching guide was to assess the use of the CAP checklists over the more traditional narrative anatomical pathology report. Participants in this work group met once a month and included the following individuals.

Georgette Haydu and Bette Smith with the Ohio Cancer Incidence Surveillance System
Pat Patterson and Mary Abbuhl with University Hospitals of Cleveland
Michele Connors with Cerner Dynamic Healthcare Technologies
Larry Derrick with Rocky Mountain Cancer Data System
Kathleen Davidson-Allen with the California Cancer Registry
Barry Gordon with C/NET Solutions
Warren Williams and Ken Gerlach with CDC-National Program of Cancer Registries

Given the different workflows used in California and Ohio, the assessment standards (or criteria) were different. These state-specific assessment standards are described in the following sections.

California

California Implementation Workflow

The following chart shows the overall California RPP implementation plan:

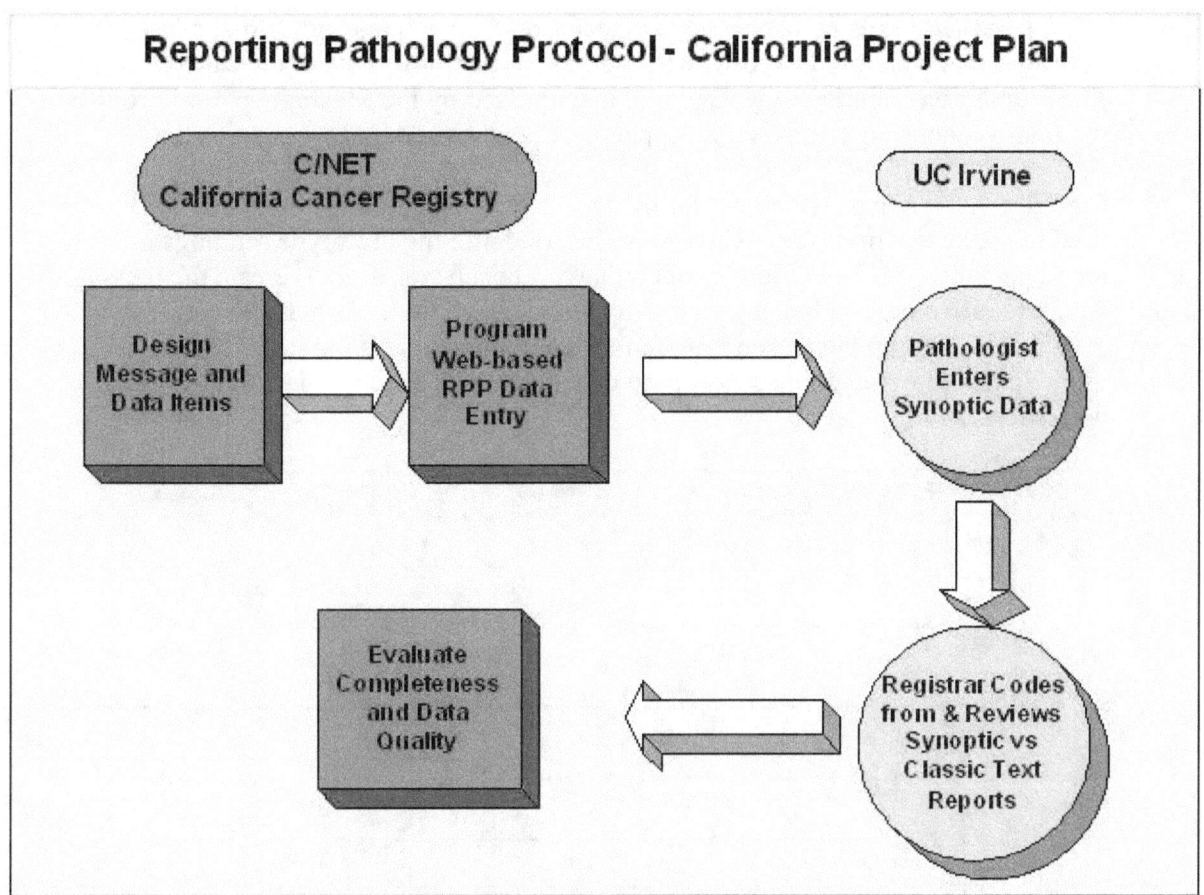

The partners involved in the California implementation were C/NET Solutions and University of California, Irvine (UCI). C/NET is a part of the Public Health Institute and provides CNExT hospital registry software to California hospitals and more than 100 others around the country. As a long-time member of Health Level 7 (HL7), C/NET staff helped the RPP messaging work group design appropriate formats and obtained Logical Observation Identifier Names and Codes (LOINC) for the checklists. CNExT software is used at the UCI registry, and future versions of that software will integrate the College of American Pathologists (CAP) Checklist data directly into registry operations. For the purposes of this pilot study, C/NET created a web-based checklist entry system to allow staff to work from different locations when creating or viewing the RPP data.

UCI has an active, research-oriented cancer registry, headed by Linda Jund, Certified Tumor Registrar (CTR). This cancer registry was very interested in helping validate the RPP colorectal checklist data for use in their registry. The Chair of UCI's Pathology Department, Fritz Lin, MD, was also interested in trying out the RPP checklists and completed the checklists for the cases in the study.

The following steps were used to carry out California's RPP implementation:

1. C/NET created implementation tables specifying the contents and format of the HL7 messages that were used to convey RPP and administrative data to the cancer registry. These tables were extensively reviewed and updated by the Messaging Workgroup and the final versions are displayed in Appendix C and Appendix D.

2. C/NET created a message object for the HL7 RPP message. This computer structure was used to create test messages, which were inserted into the prototype sending and receiving software. The Orion Symphonia workbench was used to create the message structure (see a portion below). Symphonia's message designer helps structure the CAP HL7 message components and requirements and then creates modules that can be immediately integrated into software to encode, decode, and validate the RPP HL7 messages.

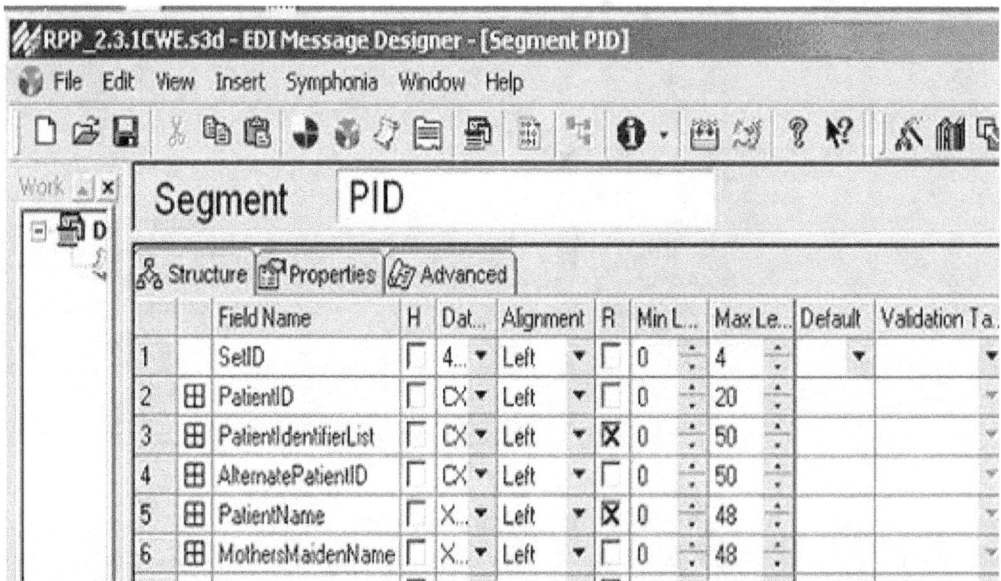

3. California carried out an exchange of test messages with Ohio/Cerner partners. Sample messages were created by using Orion's Symphonia to send to Ohio RPP partners. Synoptic messages created by Cerner were brought into the C/NET workbench to ensure there was agreement on the format implementation.

4   C/NET developed a web-based synoptic data entry system to be used by the pathologists at UCI for the three synoptic checklists. The screens were designed to look like CAP's paper-based checklists. Data captured on the screens were stored using Systematized Nomenclature of Medicine Clinical Terms (SNOMED CT) codes in an Access database. The RPP web application used secure https to protect the confidential data. (See two sections from the data entry screens below.)

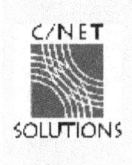

CAP Protocols - Colon and Rectum Resection

Surgical Pathology Cancer Case Summary (Checklist) Applies to invasive

carcinomas only.

College of American Pathologists

CAP January 2004; Based on AJCC/UICC TNM, 6th edition

3/16/2005

PATIENT

Name:	Anonymous , Mustbe	MedRec#:	12345678
Type of Report:	Resection	Path #: X100	Dt Collected: 3/22/05
DOB:	1/1/1800	SSN: xxx-xx-xxxx	Sex: M
Ordering MD:	Marcus Famous Welby MD	Attending MD:	Icarus Welby MD

Update Record   Signing Pathologist:

MACROSCOPIC

Specimen Type:	Right hemicolectomy
Other (specify):	
*Specimen Length:	NA cm.
Tumor Site:	Cecum
Tumor Configuration:	Infiltrative
Other (specify):	
Tumor_Size Greatest Dimension	0.5 cm.
*Dimension 2	0.5 cm.
*Dimension 3	0.2 cm.
*Mesorectum Intactness:	Not applicable

*Note: * asterisk on a field means it is not required*

5   When the web software was completed and tested, the next step was to train Dr. Lin, the Chief Pathologist at UCI, and Louella Herrmann, CTR at the UCI Hospital Cancer Registry, on how to log in and use the web site. When the pathologist completed a synoptic report, it was marked as complete and ready for viewing at the cancer registry. Because of constraints on Dr. Lin's time, he filled in paper versions of the RPP data

screens and other staff entered the data into the computer. The registry staff used the RPP web site to view the keyed data (see the evaluation section below).

California Assessment Standards and Process

In collaboration with our UCI partners, several assessments were developed to evaluate the implementation process and inclusiveness of the synoptic colon rectal checklists. The California assessments, as described below, focused on completeness, timeliness, and quality and are included as Appendix J.

The Assessment Work Group agreed to identify and use a minimum number of reports for each checklist to analyze assessments involving retrospective pathology reports. A minimum of 50 reports were to be used for the resection checklist, 5 for the local excision (transanal disk excision) checklist, and 5 for the polypectomy checklist. Starting with 2002 and working backward, the UCI cancer registry identified 50 pathology reports that were eligible for the resection checklist, 2 reports for the local excision checklist, and 0 for the polypectomy checklist. We were unable to meet the minimum number of reports for the polypectomy checklist because of the lack of invasive tumors treated only by polypectomy. The polypectomies identified were to treat either benign polyps or polyps with in situ carcinoma. We also were unable to meet the minimum requirement of five pathology reports for the local excision (transanal disk resection) checklist. Pathology reports for locally resected rectal tumors contained in situ tumors or noneligible tumors such as carcinoid tumors. Additionally, a number of cases were identified in which the local excision was performed at another institution and further surgery was performed at UCI.

Completeness
The first completeness assessment asks the question "Does the checklist provide the necessary information to code the state-required extent of disease data items?" There are three National Cancer Institute designated Surveillance, Epidemiology, and End Results (SEER) regions in California, which provide statewide coverage, so it was important to validate the ability of cancer registrars to collect the SEER extent of disease data items from the information in the checklists. The SEER extent of disease (EOD) data items were tumor size, extension of tumor, lymph node involvement (specific lymph node chain involved by tumor), number of nodes positive, and number of nodes examined.

The second completeness assessment asks the question "Is the California CAP reporting software sending all reports to the cancer registry?" (Note: This question refers to the California RPP reporting software and does not refer to a CAP software product.) To evaluate the effectiveness of the California RPP reporting software, the number of reports sent electronically was compared with the number of narrative reports identified through routine case-finding procedures for a specific time period.

The third completeness assessment asks the question "Was a checklist completed for all applicable cases?" To evaluate the completeness of reporting of all eligible cases, narrative pathology reports will be matched to their checklist counterpart.

Timeliness/Efficiency

Two assessments were developed to evaluate which format, narrative versus synoptic, is more efficient with respect to the time it takes a cancer registrar to abstract certain data items and the time it takes the pathologist to complete a pathology report. The assumption is that, if it takes less time to complete a report, the report can be available to the cancer registry sooner. Additionally, if one of the formats lends itself more readily to case abstraction, it is possible to report the case to the state registry sooner.

During the project period, hospital cancer registry staff continued to perform routine case-finding activities, which includes manually screening all pathology reports for reportable cases. To complete the first timeliness/efficiency assessment, hospital cancer registry staff measured, in minutes, the time it took to abstract certain data items from each report. All narrative reports were abstracted on one day, and all checklist reports were abstracted on another day. The data items to be abstracted included tumor size; number of lymph nodes examined; number of lymph nodes positive; histology; EOD; pathologic American Joint Committee on Cancer (AJCC) staging [Tumor (T) and Node (N) only]; margins; and lymphatic, venous, and perineural invasion.

Quality/Accuracy

Two assessments were developed for this category. The first assessment asked the question "Are the codes generated for certain data items from the SNOMED CT encoded CAP checklist as accurate as the codes produced by the cancer registry staff?"

The data entry software presents the pathologist with a drop-down box to choose the appropriate "answer" for each data element. *The International Classification of Diseases for Oncology*, 3rd edition, codes for the topography (primary site) and morphology (histologic type) are associated with the SNOMED CT CAP checklist answer codes for the tumor site and histologic type data elements. The pathologist also selects the appropriate AJCC stage for the T and N elements.

Cancer registry staff coded ICD-0-3 codes for the primary site, histology, and the AJCC T and N elements from all narrative reports for a designated period. The codes generated by the software were compared with those produced by cancer registry staff.

The second quality/accuracy assessment asked the question "Does using the checklist format enhance the quality of the data?" To answer the question, we used the 52 checklists completed for one of the above-mentioned completeness assessments to identify which data items on the checklist could not be completed with the information from the narrative pathology reports.

Additionally, we were interested in the completeness rate for the required and not-required data elements as identified for accreditation of cancer programs by the American College of Surgeons, Commission on Cancer.

California Assessment Results

The following provides the methodology and results of the evaluation assessments. As noted above, the assessments were divided into three categories: completeness, timeliness/efficiency, and quality/accuracy.

Completeness Assessments

1. Does the checklist provide the necessary information to code the state-required EOD data items?

Using the 52 narrative pathology reports identified by hospital cancer registry staff, a corresponding checklist was completed for each report. The narrative pathology reports were then reviewed and the SEER EOD data items were abstracted and coded on each report. The same procedure was performed for the completed checklists.

One hundred percent of the narrative and synoptic (checklist) pathology reports contained information to assign EOD codes. However, when the resection checklist reports were used to code the location of involved lymph nodes, there was loss of specificity for this data item because the CAP checklists do not include the name of the regional lymph node chain. The SEER EOD scheme for regional lymph node involvement of the colon and rectum are included as Appendix I. Regional lymph node chains are grouped and coded according to their relationship to the various segments of the colon, the rectosigmoid, and rectum. The coding scheme also contains a general or "NOS – Not Otherwise Specified" category.

Nineteen of the 50 narrative pathology reports contained information of metastases to the regional lymph nodes. Of these 19 reports, 11 (58%) indicated the location of the lymph nodes involved. When coding the EOD for the narrative pathology reports, a specific lymph node involvement code could be assigned for most of the applicable reports.

The colon and rectum checklists do not contain a data element to record the location of involved regional lymph nodes. Thus, the EOD lymph node involvement code "3 – Regional lymph nodes, NOS" was assigned to all resection checklists that indicated regional lymph node involvement.

In summary, both the narrative and synoptic pathology reports contain the information necessary to code SEER EOD. However, the narrative reports tend to contain detailed information to code the location of involved regional lymph nodes, whereas the CAP synoptic report format does not contain specific data elements to capture this information. The CAP Cancer Committee includes within the Checklist those concepts important for treating the patient, but this still raises the question of why regional lymph node chain name information was not included in the Checklist. The appropriateness or use of collecting regional lymph node chain name information needs to be investigated.

2. Is the reporting software sending all reports to the cancer registry?

The synoptic reports were created by using a web-based data entry software application and were completely accessible to the cancer registry. The cancer registry has the capability to review all reports online and, if necessary, to print reports.

3. Was a checklist report completed for all applicable cases?

As stated previously, the cancer registry continued the manual case-finding procedures, which includes screening all paper pathology reports and creating a suspense case in the cancer reporting software for all reportable diagnoses. For the implementation phase, the cancer registry provided the pathology department with a list of colon and rectum cancer cases they had identified through case finding that were diagnosed January 1 through September 30, 2004. The list contained the pathology report number of the specimen that initially identified a cancer diagnosis. In some instances, this was the pathology number for a biopsy. Copies of the narrative reports were provided to Dr. Fritz Lin to review and complete a checklist for all applicable reports.

Fifty-five cases were identified; however, because of time constraints, Dr. Linn was able to review only 44 narrative reports. Of the 44 reports reviewed, 21 were not eligible for a synoptic report for several reasons: (1) reports were for a biopsy only, (2) ineligible histologic types such as lymphoma and carcinoid tumors were reported, and (3) in situ tumors were reported.

Dr. Fritz Lin completed synoptic reports for 24 cases. Unfortunately, 9 cases had to be excluded from the pool for analysis because for 8 cases a synoptic report was inadvertently completed based on the biopsy specimen and not the surgical resection and 1 synoptic report was completed for an in situ carcinoma. A total of 15 cases were available to answer the first question of both the Timeliness/Efficiency and Quality/Accuracy assessments (see below).

Timeliness/Efficiency Assessments

1. Does it take less time for the cancer registrar to abstract information from the CAP checklist than from the narrative pathology report?

A form was created for the cancer registry staff to abstract the following data items from the narrative and synoptic reports for the 16 cases identified in the implementation phase:

    Tumor size
    Number of lymph nodes examined
    Number of lymph nodes positive
    Histology
    Extent of invasion (EOD)
    Pathologic AJCC staging (T and N only)
    Margins
    Lymphatic, venous, and perineural invasion.

One individual of the cancer registry staff performed this function using a stopwatch. The narrative reports were abstracted one day and the synoptic reports were done on another day. The results are depicted in the following table:

Table 1
Time to Abstract Cancer Pathology Reports in Narrative Format and Checklist Format

	Narrative Format	Checklist Format	Percent Difference
Total number of minutes to abstract all data items from 16 reports	70.57	47.54	32.6
Average number of minutes to abstract all data items from a report ($N = 16$)	4.41	2.97	32.7
Range, in minutes, to abstract all data items from 16 reports	1.50–6.40	1.27–5.33	[5]

[5] Total of eight data items from report.

The pathology report, which took more than 6 minutes to abstract, involved a discrepancy between the pathologist's and the cancer registrars' assignment of the Tumor–Node–Metastasis (TNM) stage. The checklist, which took more than 5 minutes to abstract, contained a brief statement in the preoperative findings section that caused the registrar to ponder the assignment of the codes for primary tumor (T) and distant metastasis (M).

These results show that the synoptic report resulted in an average reduction in abstracting time of more than 30%. Although we tested the synoptic report against the narrative report for only 16 cases, which required a wide range of times to abstract by either method, the results suggest that use of the synoptic method could substantially decrease abstracting time.

2. Does it take less time for the pathologist to complete the CAP checklist as opposed to a narrative pathology report?

(Note: This question refers to the California RPP reporting software and does not refer to a CAP software product.) While Dr. Fritz Lin did not use a stopwatch to measure the times, he surmised that the methods take about the same amount of time. A brief interview was conducted with Dr. Fritz Lin about his impressions of the software and the checklist format and data elements.

He thought the data entry software was well designed and he was comfortable using it; however, entering the checklist information took a fair amount of uninterrupted time.

He was concerned that the checklist format did not lend itself well to easily record cancer-related entities (adenomas, intralumenal carcinoma, dysplasia of the mucosa, etc.) and it could not be used for certain histologic types such as lymphoma and carcinoid tumors or for biopsy specimens.

He liked the uniformity of the checklist, which allows for comparative data analysis within his institution and with other institutions. Additionally, the coded data elements allow the data to be easily retrieved, which is very attractive to him.

Quality/Accuracy Assessments

1. Are the codes generated for certain data items from the CAP checklist as accurate as the codes produced by the cancer registry staff?

The abstract forms the hospital cancer staff member completed for the first Timeliness/Efficiency assessment along with the synoptic reports created by the pathologist were used to evaluate this assessment.

Three data items were assessed: primary site, histology, and AJCC staging (T and N only). Of the reports reviewed for the 15 patients, there was one discrepancy in the site assigned by the pathologist and the site assigned by the cancer registry. This was resolved during consultation with the pathologist.

The data item histologic type elicited coding discrepancies involving patients diagnosed with an Adenocarcinoma arising in an adenoma. The final diagnosis on the narrative pathology report for two cases was Adenocarcinoma arising in a tubulovillous adenoma and one case had a diagnosis of Adenocarcinoma in a tubular adenoma. *The International Classification of Diseases for Oncology*, 3rd edition (ICD-O-3), has specific morphology codes for cancers arising in different types of adenomas. Adenocarcinoma in a tubulovillous adenoma is assigned a morphology code of 8263 and Adenocarcinoma in a tubular adenoma is coded to 8210. These histologic types are not included in the checklist. All three synoptic reports contained the histologic type of Adenocarcinoma (ICDO-3 code 8140—Adenocarcinoma, NOS); however, one synoptic report contained information in the "additional pathology findings" section, which allowed the cancer registrar to assign the more specific morphology code. This finding is further discussed in the second Quality/Accuracy assessment.

Comparison of the AJCC primary tumor (T) and regional lymph nodes (N) data elements revealed one discrepancy for primary tumor and four for regional lymph nodes. Four of the five synoptic reports had an "X" value (cannot be assessed) in the T data element, whereas the cancer registry staff were able to abstract and assign a value to primary tumor. We believe this is due to the pathologist's unfamiliarity with the software application. One case had a discrepancy in the N value assigned by the pathologist and by the cancer registry due to a miscount of the number of positive lymph nodes. The pathologist assigned N1 and the cancer registry assigned N2.

2. Does using the checklist format enhance the quality of the data?

The 52 checklists completed for the above-mentioned completeness assessment were used to identify which data items on the checklist could not be completed with the information from the narrative pathology reports and to assess the completeness rate for the required and not-required data elements identified for accreditation of cancer programs by the American College of Surgeons, Commission on Cancer.

For the resection checklist, 17 required data elements and 13 not-required data elements were identified. Lists of these data elements are included in Appendix B. For the 50 colon rectum reports, 96% of the checklist data elements could be completed with the information from the narrative pathology report. The specifics on the remaining 4% are noted in the following table. The most common missing required data element was "specify margin." This was due to the surgeon failing to specify the specimen's proximal and distal margins.

Table 2
Colon and Rectum Resection Checklist
Missing Required Data Elements*
N = 50

Required Data Element	Number Unable to be Coded	Percentage
Specify Margin	11	1.3
Lymphatic Invasion (Small Vessel Invasion)	8	0.9
Venous Invasion (Large Vessel Invasion)	8	0.9
Distance Tumor From Margin	3	0.4
Radial Margin	2	0.2
Grade	1	0.1
Tumor Size	1	0.1
Proximal Margin	1	0.1
Total	35	4.0

*Note: a report can have more than one missing required data element.

Of the 50 narrative reports, 20 reports, or 40% were missing information for one or more of the checklist required data elements; thus, these checklist data elements could not be completed. Standard 4.6 of the American College of Surgeons, Commission on Cancer's Cancer Program Standards, 2004 states "The CoC [Commission on Cancer] requires that 90 percent of pathology reports that include a cancer diagnosis will contain the scientifically validated data elements outline on the surgical case summary checklist of the College of American Pathologists (CAP) publication, *Reporting on Cancer Specimens*." When this standard was applied to the 50 narrative reports reviewed, only 60% met the CoC standard.

The number of missing required data elements per narrative report ranged from nine reports missing only one required data element to one report missing four required data elements. Table 3 summarizes this information.

Table 3
Colon and Rectum Checklist
Narrative Reports Missing Required Data Elements
N = 50

Number of Missing Required Data Items	Number of Narrative Reports	Percentage
None	30	60
1	9	18
2	8	16
3	2	2
4	1	1
Total	50	100

For the 50 colon rectum reports, 63% of the not-required checklist data elements could be completed with the information from the narrative reports.

As mentioned earlier, only two narrative pathology reports were eligible for the Rectum Local Excision (transanal disk resection) Checklist. For this checklist, we identified 12 required data elements and 13 not-required data elements. All the required checklist data elements were contained in these two narrative reports. Also, we were able to complete 62% of the not-required data elements. The required and not-required data items for this checklist are included in Appendix A, Appendix G, and Appendix H.

During the process of completing a checklist for each of the 50 narrative pathology reports containing a colon resection, it was again noted that the histologic type for 8 of the 50 tumors was an adenocarcinoma arising in some type of polyp (tubular, villous, or tubulovillous). *The International Classification of Diseases for Oncology (ICDO-3)*, 3rd edition, has specific morphology codes for these types of tumors:

M-8210/3: Adenocarcinoma in tubular adenoma
M-8261/3: Adenocarcinoma in villous adenoma
M-8263/3: Adenocarcinoma in tubulovillous adenoma

In cancer registration, the basic rule for coding histology is to code the specific histologic type. The histologic type category in the colon and rectum resection checklist does not include these histologic types, but it does include the following options.

HISTOLOGIC TYPE
___ Adenocarcinoma
___ Mucinous adenocarcinoma (greater than 50% mucinous)
___ Medullary carcinoma
___ Signet-ring cell carcinoma (greater than 50% signet-ring cells)
___ Small cell carcinoma
___ Undifferentiated carcinoma
___ Other (specify): ___

____ Carcinoma, type cannot be determined

When a specimen's histology is not on the checklist, the pathologist can choose the "Other (specify)" option and then type in the more detailed histology. Participating pathologists did not use the "Other (specify)" option.

Challenges and Comments

Use of the colon and rectum checklists in the cancer registry community for case identification, data collection, research, and subsequent reporting to federal and state agencies posed several challenges. The following areas of concern were identified during the course of this project:

Case Identification

All facility-based and central registries follow standards set for tumor inclusion and reportability by one or more of the three standard setting entities: the American College of Surgeons CoC, the National Cancer Institute SEER program, and the CDC's National Program of Cancer Registries. These organizations require the inclusion of all neoplasms in the International Classification of Diseases for Oncology, Third Edition (ICD-0-3), with a behavior code of 2 or 3 (in situ or malignant), along with all nonmalignant primary intracranial and central nervous system tumors diagnosed after January 1, 2004.[6] There are a few exceptions; however, none relates to the reporting of colon and rectum tumors.

Because the colon and rectum checklists apply only to invasive cancers and exclude carcinoid tumors, lymphomas, sarcomas, tumors of the vermiform appendix, and biopsy specimens, they could not be used exclusively for case identification. They could be a welcome adjunct to the various sources used in the case-finding process and could be used as a substitute for narrative reports for those cases in which a cancer checklist exists.

Data Collection

- Regional lymph nodes containing metastatic carcinoma

Both the SEER EOD and Collaborative Staging (CS) schemas, the latter of which was implemented nationwide with cancers diagnosed on or after January 1, 2004, contain categories to code lymph node involvement based on the lymph node chain. The relevant codes are included as Appendix I.

The CAP Resection and Local Excision Colon and Rectum Checklists allow for recording the number of lymph nodes examined and the number involved with cancer as well as assigning either AJCC N1 or N2, which denotes regional lymph node involvement. However, the checklists do not contain a discrete data element for the lymph node chain involved with cancer (e.g., ileocolic, inferior mesenteric). Regional lymph node chains are grouped and coded

---

[6] North American Association of Central Cancer Registries: Standards for Cancer Registries, Volume II: Data Standards and Data Dictionary, Tenth Edition, Chapter III.

according to their relationship to the various segments of the colon, the rectosigmoid, and the rectum. Without this information, the SEER EOD lymph node data items would be coded 3 for "Regional Lymph Nodes" as opposed to 1 or 2 for a more specific named lymph node chain. Both checklists contain a "comments" area where this information can be recorded. Whether this affects cancer registration and treatment provided by clinicians requires additional study.

- Specific morphology codes

As noted earlier, a number of resection specimens contain Adenocarcinoma arising in some type of adenoma (tubular, villous, or tubulovillous). The code set used by all cancer registries nationwide and contained in *The International Classification of Diseases for Oncology*, 3rd edition (ICD-O-3), contain specific morphology codes for these types of tumors.

The histologic type section of the colon rectum resection checklist does not include a category for these specific histologic entities. To capture this detailed information on histologic type, one could use the "Adenocarcinoma" category and include details about the adenoma in the comments section or use the "Other (specify)" category. Per the cancer registry coding rules, the more specific histology code is required.

Ohio

Ohio Implementation Workflow

The Ohio RPP was designed as collaboration between the Ohio Department of Health's (ODH) cancer registry, the Ohio Cancer Incidence Surveillance System (OCISS); the pathologists at the University Hospitals of Cleveland (UHC); UHC's software vendor, Cerner Dynamic Healthcare Technologies, Inc. (Cerner); and the OCISS database software vendor Rocky Mountain Cancer Data Systems (RMCDS). The objective of the project was to develop a computer program for use by pathologists, based on the colon and rectum cancers Systematized Nomenclature of Medicine Clinical Terms (SNOMED CT) encoded College of American Pathologists (CAP) checklists and to transfer the data in a Health Level 7 (HL7) format to the central registry. OCISS found this to be a practical approach that would result in a system model that pathology laboratories could use in any setting, hospital or free-standing, to submit data directly to a state's central cancer registry.

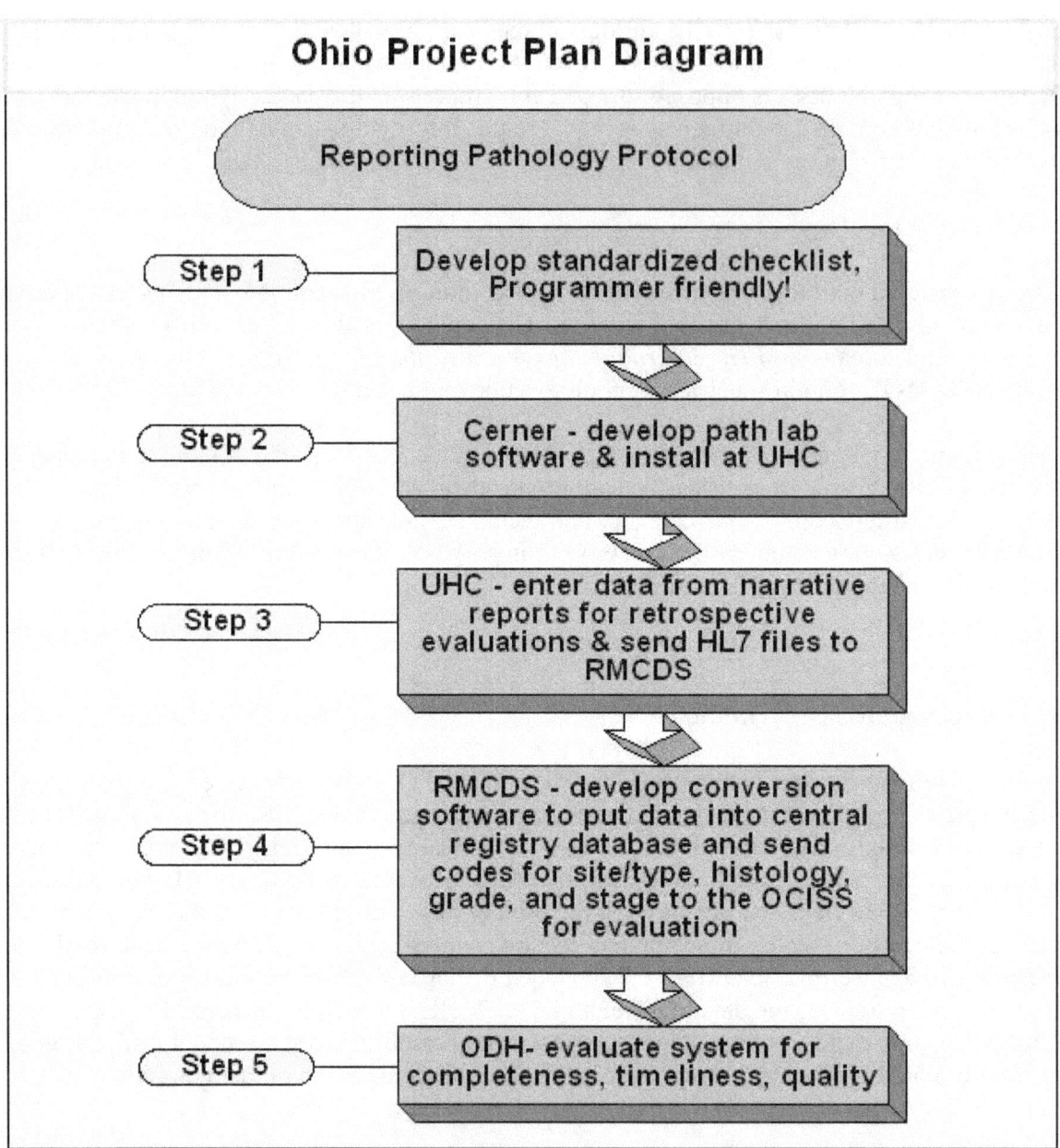

The diagram above describes the work plan for the project, which occurred in the five, chronologically overlapping steps described below.

Step 1: RPP participants from Ohio, California, and CDC-National Program of Cancer Registries (NPCR) worked with CAP and SNOMED International to translate the SNOMED CT encoded CAP colorectal checklist into an HL7 message. Working out the details of how the CAP cancer checklists should be represented online was a challenge. For more information about this process, see the section Messaging Work Group.

As noted in the Messaging Work Group section, every item on each CAP checklist had to be coded, and in some cases that meant adding new data items and defining new codes in the Cerner CoPathPlus system and including them in the worksheet definitions. In addition, the CoPathPlus HL7 results interface had to be enhanced to include the new synoptic coded data, plus other fields such as ordering provider name, facility, address, and phone that were not in the Cerner standard results interface.

Step 2: Cerner had already developed a synoptic reporting module for the CoPathPlus anatomic pathology information system. This module provided tools for building online "worksheets" that follow the layout of the CAP cancer checklists. Cerner also had the ability to produce HL7 results interface messages, but these did not include the coded synoptic data that are the key to this project. Enhancing the "front end" software for entering the SNOMED CT coded cancer checklists and enhancing the "back end" software to produce the specified HL7 messages were the focus of Cerner's involvement in the RPP project.

The synoptic reporting module resulting from Step 1 activities were installed at University Hospitals' pathology laboratory. Users were trained to use the module, and the latest versions of the colorectal worksheets were loaded. Updates to the worksheets were necessary as the CAP checklists and message specifications evolved.

Step 3: UHC provided consultation for pathology-related coding issues and, during this step, provided the information used to evaluate the system by entering data from narrative pathology reports. Dr. Joseph Willis, an ardent supporter of the need for standardization within the pathology laboratory, entered data for 76 colon and rectum surgical specimens from narrative reports into the checklist via the computerized synoptic reporting module developed by Cerner.

Step 4: RMCDS provided central registry software expertise. Cerner had worked out the means to transport the output messages, containing protected patient information, from University Hospitals to RMCDS in the HL7 format. This simple step took some time to work out to ensure that Health Insurance Portability and Accountability Act of 1996 regulations and patient confidentiality concerns were met. Briefly, UHC could not release data directly to RMCDS; however, the data could be transmitted to OCISS.

Step 5: OCISS provided Certified Tumor Registrar expertise in coding cancer data and in evaluating the accuracy of the translation of critical data items using the new project system as well as administrative and coordinating functions. In addition, OCISS evaluated the new system as described below and in the appendices.

Ohio Assessment Standards and Process

Below is an overview of the evaluation measures in Ohio.

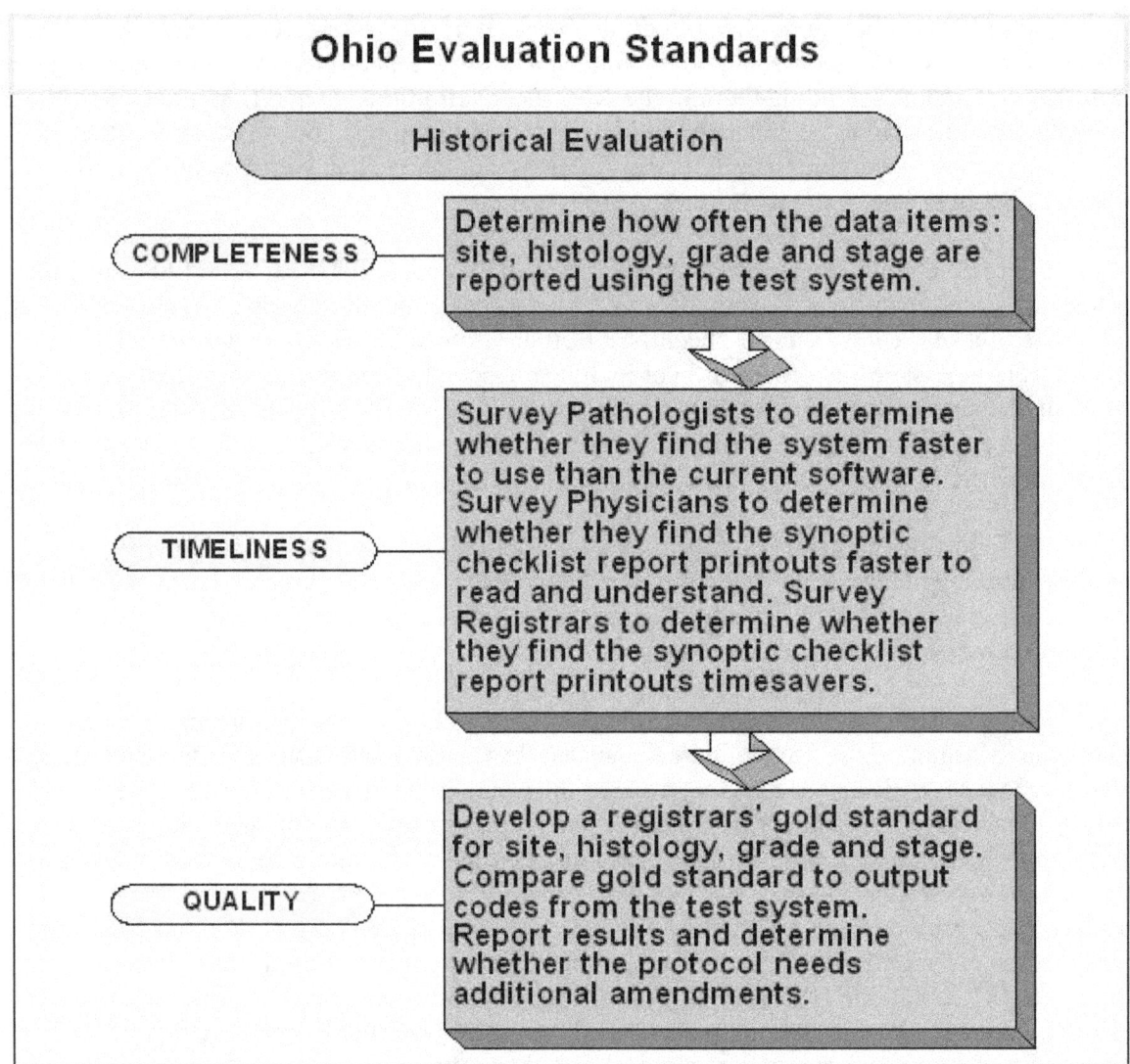

The complete Ohio RPP Evaluation Measurers is included in Appendix K. The objective of this evaluation is to determine the quality (or accuracy), completeness, and timeliness of reporting cancer with the checklist system developed as a result of efforts of the RPP conducted in Ohio.

OCISS received narrative pathology reports for 76 cases of colorectal cancer. The pathologist at UHC entered the data from the original narrative pathology reports into the checklist system developed for the RPP project. Of the 76 specimens, 69 were from resections, 4 were from local excisions, and 3 were from polypectomies.

Pathology data being evaluated were entered into the synoptic checklist system and downloaded from UHC in HL7 message format on three different occasions during the project period and were electronically transmitted to RMCDS, which converted each batch into a North American Association of Central Cancer Registries (NAACCR) Volume II format and printed a line listing with the medical record number for each case along with the codes for site, histology, grade, and stage. RMCDS sent the line listings to OCISS to compare with the codes generated by OCISS registrars' reviews and abstracts of the original narrative reports. A Microsoft Excel file was constructed to record the codes generated by each method, OCISS, and checklist. OCISS staff then tallied how often the OCISS and checklist codes were not in agreement (i.e., nonmatches) and how often the checklist codes were left blank when the OCISS codes were not left blank (where both were left blank, a match was indicated as information might be unavailable in the narrative).

Ohio's evaluation was designed to test how well the system was able to translate, code, and transmit four of the most critical data items in the pathology report: site, histology, stage, and grade. The first three items are especially important to a state cancer registry charged with surveillance as they are essential for calculating rates of cancer. Grade is of special importance to physicians and patients as it is important in determining the most appropriate treatment.

As noted above, completeness, timeliness, and quality of the data were assessed in this evaluation.

Completeness was determined according to whether all four data items are transmitted in their entirety—i.e., there are no blanks.

Timeliness is a major reason for the interest that central registries have in developing the capacity for pathology laboratories to report cancers electronically. With a pathology laboratory reporting all cancers electronically, the potential exists for cancer registries to receive such reports almost immediately and thus allow for measures of incidence to be produced earlier than the 2 to 3 years now required. Although this aspect of timeliness is of interest, it is not the intent or within the scope of this project to measure that aspect of timeliness.

For this project, timeliness is measured in three ways. First, pathologist review of the checklist system will be used to determine whether the time to use the checklist in the laboratory setting would encourage its use in practice. Because implementation of this pilot project cannot replace the routine in the pathology laboratory at UHC, a timed trial is not possible. Therefore, the pathologist's opinion about timeliness will be the measure used after he or she has used the system to enter data from narrative reports.

The other two aspects of timeliness will be to obtain the opinions of cancer registrars and physicians who will assess the printed report from the checklist system and to obtain their opinions about whether this type of report will save them time. The UHC Surgical Pathology Report (the "synoptic checklist report printout" referred to in the diagram above) in the appendix is the report produced by the computerized checklist system. It features a well organized CAP Tumor Summary on the first page that lists information on Specimen Type, Tumor Site, Tumor Configuration, Tumor Size, Intactness of Mesorectum, Histologic Type, Histologic Grade, Pathology Staging TNM, Margins, Lymphatic Invasion, Venous Invasion, Perineural Invasion, Tumor Border Configuration, Tumoral Lymphocytic Response, and Additional Pathologic Findings. This is followed by the narrative pathology report. This well-organized summary of the most pertinent, standardized medical information displayed on the first page may prove to be a time-saver for physicians and cancer registrars.

Quality will be determined by comparing the codes for the four critical data items (site, histology, stage, and grade) in the checklist system (i.e., the codes that are transmitted to the cancer registry) with the codes that expert registrars abstracted and coded from the original narrative pathology reports on which the checklist data are based.

In Ohio's implementation of the project, data entered into the computerized checklist system by the pathologist at UHC were converted into an HL7 file, which then had to be transmitted and converted into an RMCDS database file in a NAACCR format. This involved three processes: use of the checklist input software in the pathology laboratory, conversion of the input data into an HL7 message, and RMCDS conversion of the HL7 message into the NAACCR Volume II format. Thus, difficulties in programming have to be traced to their source among these processes.

In later stages of this project, OCISS staff members came up with some questions about what might be called "knowledge, attitudes, and beliefs" concerning standardized pathology reporting. To get a feel for the answers, OCISS registrars asked a few of their colleagues to show the SNOMED CT encoded CAP checklist to some of their hospitals' physicians and pathologists and request their opinions about the report and about standardized pathology laboratory reporting in general. Four hospital cancer registrars were also asked for their opinions of this report, from which hospital and patient identifiers had been removed. They were also asked to conduct a short survey interview with a few of the physicians and/or pathologists (see surveys in appendices) at their hospitals after showing them the SNOMED CT encoded CAP Checklist and a blank copy of the synoptic checklist report printout.

Two of the reporting source registrars showed the SNOMED CT encoded CAP Checklist to three pathologists at their facilities and asked them to assess two statements: (1) "I like the idea of standardizing pathology data to make it more useful for physicians, researchers, and cancer registries"; and (2) "As long as the narrative is still part of the record, I would be willing to adapt my procedures for capturing analytic data to include this type of checklist (either in a paper or electronic format)." They were asked to answer based on a five-point scale from strongly disagree to strongly agree. Two of the three "strongly agreed" with both questions and one "agreed." All three of them were from the same American College of Surgeons (ACoS)-approved facility. It would be interesting to know more about the openness of pathologists in non-ACoS hospitals to this type of development.

All four volunteer reporting source registrars showed the synoptic checklist report printout to physicians at their hospitals. Eight physicians registered opinions on standardized pathology reporting. Four of the eight 'Strongly Agreed' that they preferred the standardized checklist type of report and two 'Agreed'. The other two 'Did Not Know'. Three of the eight 'Strongly Agreed' that the standardized report with the checklist type summary at the beginning would save them time and three 'Agreed', whereas one 'Did Not Know' and one 'Disagreed'.

Ohio Assessment Results

Completeness

Completeness was defined as the extent to which all data items were received by the state registry for site, histology, grade, and stage (T and N) data items (i.e., 5 data items) for each of the 76 cases for which data were submitted for a total of 370 data items. Ohio did not include the M or metastasis portion of the staging data being evaluated because pathology laboratories usually do not have complete information about metastatic status.

Review of the 76 case reports for which data were received from UHC using the electronic checklist system and comparing those data with abstracts of the original narrative reports for those 76 cases showed data to be 99.2% (367/370) complete when the checklist system was used for transmitting the data. Three data items were submitted with blanks. One blank appeared for histology, where a large cell neuroendocrine tumor was diagnosed, but the histology code did not get transmitted. The histologic type concept in the checklist contains seven histologies with an additional choice of "Other (specify)." Neuroendocrine tumor (8246/3) is not included in the core seven histologies and therefore must be entered in the "Other (specify)" category as text. Because this is text, there is no associated code in the SNOMED CT encoded CAP Checklist or the message. Two blanks for stage correspond to unknown stage coded by OCISS registrars. These could be eliminated if the software program included a feature that requires that all selections take place before proceeding to the next record or by developing an intrafield edit to ensure that blanks are not transmitted for all essential (or required) data items. Because they represented unknowns, the blanks for stage were considered to be accurate for purposes of assessing quality below, however.

Timeliness

The pathologists' opinion about the timeliness of incorporating a checklist-type system into the workflow within the setting of the pathology laboratory is an important part of this evaluation. It was first necessary to understand the workflow. This became clear during a site visit to UHC's pathology laboratory when Dr. Willis and his surgical pathology team demonstrated the process, as follows: (1) a member of the surgical pathology team grossly examines the specimen "at the bench" and dictates the specimen gross description; (2) he or she then submits to the histology laboratory representative sections of the tissue to be processed for microscopic examination; (3) next, a transcriptionist enters gross specimen dictation into the laboratory computer system to generate the working draft of the pathology report; (4) later, the surgical pathology team member examines the slides at the microscope, sitting beside the computer where he or she dictates the microscopic information to generate the final diagnosis in narrative form on the report.

To use a computerized checklist system, instead of dictating additional microscopic information while examining slides, the pathologist would simply select answers from the checklist based on information from the transcription and what he or she sees on the slides. Dr. Willis believes that, although it would require a change in procedure and, accordingly, some adjustment, using the checklist probably would not take any longer than dictating information during the microscopic examination. The change in procedure could involve pathologists using an electronic system such as a computer during the examination instead of dictating their impressions during microscopic examination. He strongly endorses the importance of explicitly recording the CAP standardized data in this manner.

Another measure of timeliness used was a survey of the opinions of cancer registrars and physicians as to whether the synoptic checklist report printout would save time. This report organizes the pertinent, standardized medical information on cancer site, histology, stage, and grade in the CAP summary section on the front page where it is easy to find.

Saving time for registrars: Four Ohio hospital registrars were surveyed using the instrument shown in Appendix M, after reviewing deidentified copies of the synoptic checklist report printout pathology report also shown in Appendix N. All the registrars agreed that the "College of American Pathologists Summary" at the beginning of the University of Hospitals of Cleveland Surgical Pathology Report would save time abstracting data for the hospital registry.

In addition, all OCISS registrars who have reviewed the synoptic checklist report printout agree that this type of report would save time in instances when they must rely on paper copies to visually review information. This may be important when electronic transfer of data-item-specific information from the pathology laboratory is not possible or when paper reports are preferable.

Saving time for physicians: In a survey (see Appendix L) conducted by OCISS registrars, four Ohio hospital registrars shared the synoptic checklist report printout with eight physicians in their hospitals. The physicians were asked to assess two statements on a five-point scale from "strongly agree" to "strongly disagree." One statement was that "This report might save time." Only one physician disagreed, perhaps because his hospital already had a very structured report. One did not know if this type of report would save time, again, perhaps because his hospital already had a fairly structured report. Six of the eight physicians either agreed ($N = 3$) or strongly agreed ($N = 3$) that this type of printed report with a very structured summary of information collected with the checklist approach would save them time. It may be inferred from this small sample that physicians believe time could be saved by using a system that produces a report with a standardized and structured summary conveniently placed at the beginning. Further study is needed to corroborate this in a more concrete manner.

Quality (Accuracy)

Accuracy was evaluated based on the logic that the codes used by cancer registries for critical data items (site, histology, stage, and grade) should be the same whether abstracted by certified cancer registrars from the original narrative report or received through the checklist system in which the coding starts with the pathologist selecting from the standardized checklist and then is fully automated and transferred into the registry database. Therefore, the evaluation compares the codes abstracted by certified cancer registrars, used as the gold standard, from the original narrative reports with the codes produced by the checklist system.

The percent of Checklist data matching the OCISS "gold standard" data is as follows:

	Site	Histology	Grade	Stage	Total
Total	76	76	76	76	304
Non-match	12	20	2	10	47
Match	61	56	74	66	257
% Matching	86.5	73.7	97.4	86.8	84.5

Site: For site, 86.5%, or 61 cases matched.
The table below indicates the discrepancies between the site codes abstracted by OCISS registrars from the original pathology reports and those reported by the pathology laboratory from the checklist system.

Case	OCISS	Checklist	Reason for Discrepancy
		Non-matching OCISS/Checklist Site Codes	
1	C18.2 ascending colon	C18.9 colon NOS	Registrar more specific
2	C18.2 ascending colon	C18.9 colon NOS	Registrar more specific
3	C18.7 sigmoid colon	C18.9 colon NOS	Registrar more specific
4	C18.4 transverse colon	C18.9 colon NOS	Registrar more specific
5	C18.7 sigmoid colon	C18.9 colon NOS	Registrar more specific
6	C18.9 colon NOS	C18.2 ascending colon	Pathologist more specific
7	C18.9 colon NOS	C18.7 sigmoid colon	Pathologist more specific
8	C18.9 colon NOS	C18.7 sigmoid colon	Pathologist more specific
9	C18.0 cecum	C18.2 ascending colon	Coding error
10	C20.9 rectum	C18.7 sigmoid colon	Coding error
11	C19.9 rectosigmoid junction	C18.7 sigmoid colon	Coding error
12	C18.0 cecum	C18.2 ascending colon	Ambiguity in pathology report text

Note: NOS = not otherwise specified.

As shown in the table above, of the 76 cases reported using the checklist system, 64 of the site codes matched those abstracted by OCISS registrars for a score of 86.5% matching. For 8 of the 12 cases for which reported site did not match the OCISS abstracted site, the reported checklist site code was less specific in five instances and more specific in three instances. Of the remaining 4 non-matches, 3 were due to errors in coding as determined by a senior OCISS registrar who performed a blind review of the original pathology laboratory report to determine what the correct coding should be. To avoid bias in determining the correct coding, the senior registrar was not made aware of which code was abstracted by OCISS registrars and which was assigned with the checklist. The last non-matched case occurred because of ambiguities in the narrative text of the original pathology report according to the senior registrar.

Histology: For histology, 73.7%, or 56 cases matched.

Non-matching OCISS/Checklist Histology Codes		
Case	OCISS	Checklist
1	8263/3 Adenocarcinoma in tubulovillous adenoma	8480/3 Mucinous Adenocarcinoma
2	8263/3 Adenocarcinoma in tubulovillous adenoma	8140/3 Adenocarcinoma
3	8263/3 Adenocarcinoma in tubulovillous adenoma	8140/3 Adenocarcinoma
4	8263/3 Adenocarcinoma in tubulovillous adenoma	8140/3 Adenocarcinoma
5	8480/3 Mucinous Adenocarcinoma	8140/3 Adenocarcinoma
6	8263/3 Adenocarcinoma in tubulovillous adenoma	8140/3 Adenocarcinoma
7	8480/3 Mucinous Adenocarcinoma	8140/3 Adenocarcinoma
8	8210/3 Adenocarcinoma in adenomatous polyp	8140/3 Adenocarcinoma
9	8263/3 Adenocarcinoma in tubulovillous adenoma	8140/3 Adenocarcinoma
10	8263/3 Adenocarcinoma in tubulovillous adenoma	8140/3 Adenocarcinoma
11	8480/3 Mucinous Adenocarcinoma	8140/3 Adenocarcinoma
12	8210/3 Adenocarcinoma in adenomatous polyp	8140/3 Adenocarcinoma
13	8480/3 Mucinous Adenocarcinoma	8140/3 Adenocarcinoma
14	8210/3 Adenocarcinoma in adenomatous polyp	8140/3 Adenocarcinoma
15	8013/3 Large cell neuroendocrine carcinoma	Blank
16	8261/3 Adenocarcinoma in villous adenoma	8140/3 Adenocarcinoma
17	8263/3 Adenocarcinoma in tubulovillous adenoma	8140/3 Adenocarcinoma
18	8210/3 Adenocarcinoma in adenomatous polyp	8140/3 Adenocarcinoma
19	8263/3 Adenocarcinoma in tubulovillous adenoma	8140/3 Adenocarcinoma
20	8480/3 Mucinous Adenocarcinoma	8140/3 Adenocarcinoma

The HL7 message for histology as received from RMCDS by Ohio's registry included two codes, 8140/3 (Adenocarcinoma, NOS) in 74 instances and 8480/3 (Mucinous adenocarcinoma) in 2 instances. OCISS registrars coded 8263/3 (Adenocarcinoma in tubulovillous adenoma), 8261/3 (Adenocarcinoma in villous adenoma), and 8210/3 (Adenocarcinoma in adenomatous polyp) as well. In five cases, the pathologist used the Adenocarcinoma code (8140/3), whereas the OCISS registrars used the Mucinous Adenocarcinoma code (8480/3). The Checklist Histologic Type section pertaining to Mucinous Adenocarcinoma contains the limitation of "greater than 50% Mucinous": "___ Mucinous adenocarcinoma (greater than 50% mucinous)". Histologic Type coding rules for the cancer registry community as noted in The *SEER Program Code Manual*[7] state, "Code the histologic type using the following rules in sequence" and "B. the more specific term if one is an 'NOS' term (carcinoma) and the other term is more specific." Therefore, it appears that there was a discrepancy between the coding rules used by pathologists and those used by cancer registrars.

The number of histologies included in the CAP colorectal cancer checklist is limited to a choice of seven (see below). There are dozens of possible histologies for colorectal cancers. If the tumor is a specific type not offered on the checklists, the pathologist may select "Other, specify." As noted earlier, the histology with the blank code was the large cell neuroendocrine tumor and is an example of the use of the "Other (specify)" option. Neuroendocrine tumor (8246/3) is not included in the core seven histologies (see below) and therefore must be entered in the "Other (specify)" category as text. Because this is text, there is no associated code in the SNOMED CT encoded CAP Checklist or the message. In such circumstances, cancer registries must find another way to code the associated text. This problem needs to be resolved in programming the checklist, perhaps by including a complete selection of histology choices for colorectal cancers.

Checklist Choices (January 2004):	Corresponding
HISTOLOGIC TYPE	Histology Code
Adenocarcinoma	8140/3
___ Mucinous adenocarcinoma (greater than 50% mucinous)	8480/3
Medullary carcinoma	8510/3
Signet-ring cell carcinoma (greater than 50% signet-ring cells)	8490/3
Small cell carcinoma	8041/3
Undifferentiated carcinoma	8020/3
Other (specify):	Not coded
Carcinoma, type cannot be determined	8010/3

Grade: For grade, 97.4%, or 74 cases matched.

For two cases grade was coded as "NO-Re," RMCDS notation for "No-Recode." Discussion with RMCDS revealed that this has the same meaning as the checklist item "Cannot be assessed" or "Grade cannot be determined." This concept should have been converted, in the grade data item, to "9" for "Grade/differentiation unknown, not stated, or not applicable." In both cases, the OCISS registrars abstracted a code of 9, unknown, which would have agreed with the checklist

---

[7] The *SEER Program Code Manual*, 3rd edition p. 96

data had the coding been converted correctly. The conversion program at the central registry needs to be adjusted.

Stage: For stage, 84.5%, or 66 cases matched.

As noted earlier, OCISS collects stage information relying on the AJCC Cancer Staging Manual, Sixth Edition, or the TNM schema. There is a corresponding section in the CAP cancer checklists for T, N, and M. Below is the AJCC TNM schema for colon and rectum cancers. Note that, in the CAP Cancer Checklists, the Distant Metastasis (M) list does not include the M0 code, no distant metastasis. Because pathologists are working only with the specimen, they cannot definitively make a statement of no distant metastasis.

Primary Tumor (T)

TX	Primary tumor cannot be assessed
T0	No evidence of primary tumor
Tis	Carcinoma in situ: intraepithelial or invasion of lamina propria
T1	Tumor invades submucosa
T2	Tumor invades muscularis propria
T3	Tumor invades through the muscularis propria into the subserosa, or into non-peritonealized pericolic or perirectal tissues
T4	Tumor directly invades other organs or structures, and/or perforates visceral peritoneum

Regional Lymph Nodes (N)

NX	Regional lymph nodes cannot be assessed
N0	No regional lymph node metastasis
N1	Metastasis in 1 to 3 regional lymph nodes
N2	Metastasis in 4 or more regional lymph

Distant Metastasis (M)

MX	Cannot be assessed
M0	No distant metastasis
M1	Distant metastasis

In the CAP checklists, in addition to the above items, there are some extra codes as noted below. Asterisks indicate that the codes are optional. These codes are not part of the AJCC TNM Manual, but they are part of the *TNM Supplement. A Commentary on Uniform Use*, 2nd edition, and are included in a chapter entitled "Optional Proposals for Testing New Telescopic Ramifications of TNM."

*___ pT3a/b: Tumor invades through the muscularis propria into the subserosa or the nonperitonealized pericolic or perirectal soft tissues, invades 5 mm or less beyond the border of the muscularis propria
*___ pT3c/d: Tumor invades through the muscularis propria into the subserosa or the nonperitonealized pericolic or perirectal soft tissues, invades greater than 5 mm beyond the border of the muscularis propria

These optional codes were used by the UHC Pathology Laboratory and were transported in the associated message a total of 18 times. OCISS staff were not expecting two digits in this data item. In those circumstances the "a/b" codes were dropped to be consistent with the OCISS database system, and the AJCC TNM Manual, 6th Edition. Ideally, the conversion program from the HL7 message to the cancer registry database should have dropped these letter codes.

After the "a/b" codes were dropped, there were 10 remaining nonmatches as shown in the table below:

Non-matching OCISS/Checklist Stage Codes					
Case ID	OCISS		Checklist		Number of Discrepancies
	T	N	T	N	
1	2	0	3	0	1
2	3	1	4	1	1
3	3	1	4	1	1
4	3	2	4	2	1
5	2	0	3	0	1
6	3	2	4	2	1
7	3	1	4	1	1
8	3	2	2	1	2
9	3	1	4	1	1
Total Discrepancies					10

Discrepancies in the codes for stage between the pathologist's interpretation and the registrar's interpretation of the narrative text involve whether invasion of the tumor actually penetrates through the muscularis propria into the subserosa or perforates the visceral peritoneum. However, it must be noted that this is an assessment of the "discrepancies between interpretations" of the narrative text and not discrepancies caused by a problem in the checklist or in the computerized programs developed by Cerner or by RMCDS for the transfer of data to OCISS.

Ohio's Challenges and Comments

Ohio's project team assisted with developing the HL7 message structure for the CAP checklist concepts, developed an input program for use by the participating pathology team, entered a limited number of cancer reports into that program, converted the data to the agreed upon HL7 message, and transmitted the information in the HL7 message to the RMCDS who converted the HL7 messages into standard cancer registry data item format. The evaluation reported here was conducted in one stage looking critically at data entering the registry database. It did not measure each step in the process separately (the checklist, the Cerner software, the HL7 message, and the RMCDS conversion), which might be advisable in a fully documented assessment.

Completeness was measured at 99.2% in terms of measuring that all four critical data items were completely transmitted by the checklist system, including the software at the pathology laboratory and the entire system for transmitting data from the pathology laboratory in an HL7 messaging system to RMCDS and conversion into the NAACCR format and into the OCISS database. A minor adjustment in the software could bring this up to 100%.

There are several ways to look at timeliness in relation to pathology laboratory data. First, one may look at the pathologist's time. It was not possible to do actual timed studies to see if using the checklist system takes the pathologist more or less time than the current procedure. The pathologist was simply asked for an opinion about the impact of using the system on his time. OCISS also asked others who would be using the products of the pathologist's use of the checklist, the physicians and the cancer registrars, to look at the standardized, printed pathology reports to see if they might represent a saving of time for them. Another aspect of timeliness that could have been measured to assess the value of instituting a checklist system is faster entry of case data into the state cancer registry. OCISS finds that some cases are not reported for many months and hopes that standardized laboratory reporting might help to increase timeliness in this respect as well.

One aspect of completeness and timeliness not addressed in this assessment is the overall timeliness of reporting to the cancer registry that might allow for surveillance earlier than at 24 months. The pathology laboratory data could also be used for case-finding purposes to identify cases not being reported by other facilities that should be reporting them. It is necessary to provide a streamlined computerized system for doing this to facilitate such a function, but with the checklist in use by pathologists, this might become a possibility.

As for the quality or accuracy of the data, the evaluation showed significant discrepancies (only 84.5% agreement overall) between the pathologist and the registrars' "gold standard" (often a negotiated value). It is very important to note that neither the checklist nor the software appears to be a problem here. The differences appear to be differences in interpretation of the narrative report. This area of assessment is difficult, as it begs the question of whose interpretation is correct, especially in light of the fact that neither pathologist nor registrar was looking at a specimen, but both parties were interpreting a narrative report—sometimes many months after the fact. This may be a side effect of the pilot project and should not be an issue when pathologists are using the CAP checklists as part of the routine processing of cancer pathology reports. We believe this assessment unexpectedly demonstrated the importance of getting information directly from the pathologist interpreting directly from the specimen instead of relying on someone else interpreting from a narrative report at a later date—a good argument in favor of checklist development and use in the laboratory setting.

Overall recommendations for the Ohio team are as follows:
1. The checklist needs to include all histology codes as choices in the Other category.
2. Checklist software should not allow for blanks.
3. There was a steep learning curve as people from various backgrounds adjusted to one another's vocabularies and intellectual perspectives to develop a basis for establishing consensus. It is highly recommended that future projects seek to build on this foundation as much as possible instead of starting over each time.

Discussion and Conclusions

This project required a considerable amount of time to allow for a process of acculturation among team members. Because of the nature of the project, expertise had to be drawn from several highly specialized fields: cancer registration, pathology, anatomical pathology laboratory management, laboratory information systems, the CAP Cancer Checklists, and the SNOMED CT vocabulary. People in specialized fields develop specialized languages and unique perspectives; therefore, it took time to develop a common language and to widen viewpoints to establish the kind of communication needed to move RPP ahead, particularly with regard to fine points of messaging and coding and finding common ground between the needs of pathologists and the needs of cancer registrars. The CAP checklist and the HL7 message standards were new tools for most team members, which added to the learning curve. All these aspects of project development were necessary and time-consuming but essential to the success of the effort. The RPP team, in effect, had to develop the ability to think in common terms from a common perspective using new tools before moving toward project goals.

Checklists
Within the CAP Cancer Checklists, there are required (or essential) data items and not-required (non-essential) data items. For this pilot project, all data items were collected. From one perspective, the CAP checklist data items represent the basis of part of an anatomical pathology laboratory surveillance or research database. Some of the data items from the CAP checklist are directly mappable into the cancer registry database, but others are not. An issue for future submissions of the CAP cancer checklist data to cancer registries is to determine whether the cancer registry system should collect and maintain all or a portion of the CAP checklist data items.

During the course of this project, participants encountered a number of other (non-CAP) cancer pathology synoptic or checklist reports. In addition to CAP, several other organizations have developed cancer pathology checklist reports. From a national cancer surveillance perspective, a multitude of cancer pathology checklists is a concern. For the cancer surveillance community, the CAP Cancer Checklists are the national standard. The American College of Surgeons (ACoS) Commission on Cancer (CoC) hospital program standard 4.6[8] states: "The CoC requires that 90 percent of pathology reports that include a cancer diagnosis will contain the scientifically validated data elements outlined on the surgical case summary checklist of the College of American Pathologists (CAP) publication, reporting on Cancer Specimens." The SNOMED CT encoded CAP Cancer Checklists offer the added advantage of providing standardized codes for these concepts. The use of these enhanced checklists could promote national implementation of cancer pathology reports containing discrete data item information.

There is an associated license fee for commercial use of the CAP Cancer Checklists and for the use of the SNOMED CT encoded version of the Checklists, but that fee seems relatively reasonable especially when compared with the licensing fee for the associated software from the anatomical pathology laboratory information system (LIS) vendors. The associated software development costs are passed onto the anatomical pathology laboratory. So while computerized versions of the CAP Cancer Checklists may be more desirable, they are also more expensive, at least initially.

---

[8] Commission on Cancer, *Cancer Program Standards 2004*, p. 38

The CAP checklists provide a set of core data items, essential and non-essential. Individual laboratories and hospitals, however, will want to add new concepts to the checklist to meet the unique needs of the institution. The issue remains as to how local or additional customized concepts should be handled in the HL7 message, if at all and how cancer registries should handle that information.

The checklists were originally designed as paper forms and not as software. The checklist data items could form the basis of an anatomical pathology laboratory database. The checklist paper form was able to capture (through indentation) whether more than one item could be checked because at times a subtype of a checked item could also be chosen. The following example from the polypectomy checklist shows that a choice of "Uninvolved by invasive carcinoma" leads to a second question (or sub-question), "Distance of invasive carcinoma from margin: ___ mm." The second set of information, "Distance of invasive carcinoma from margin: ___ mm" is required only if the prior option, "Uninvolved by invasive carcinoma," is checked. The information inherent in the formatting of the paper form had to be translated into appropriate business rules and the associated software design.

Polypectomy Checklist Example:
"MARGINS (check all that apply)

Deep margin (Stalk margin)
___ Cannot be assessed
___ Uninvolved by invasive carcinoma
     Distance of invasive carcinoma from margin: ___ mm
___ Involved by invasive carcinoma"

As with any set of industry national standards, the checklists will evolve. The CAP Cancer Checklists are updated once a year, in January, whereas SNOMED CT is released twice a year, in January and July. Therefore, a limited number of the SNOMED CT codes could change in the July and January release due to changes in the terminology, whereas the CAP un-encoded Checklists would only potentially change on a yearly basis. This issue of including the date of the SNOMED CT encoded checklist version within the HL7 message is also discussed under the following Messaging section heading.

Some of these updates warrant considerable changes to associated software systems. For example, during the course of the project, the following concept from the Colon and Rectum: Resection Checklist was changed to clarify the intent of the CAP Cancer Committee.

Resection Checklist Example:
*MESORECTUM
*___ Not applicable *[F-02B8F, 384611000] Invasion of mesorectum by tumor not applicable (finding)*
*___ Complete *[R-00409, 384608001] complete invasion of mesorectum by tumor (finding)*
*___ Near complete *[R-0040A, 384609009] Near complete invasion of mesorectum by tumor (finding)*
*___ Incomplete *[R-0040B, 384610004] incomplete invasion of mesorectum by tumor (finding)*

The above section was replaced with the following section.

Resection Checklist Example:

*INTACTNESS OF MESORECTUM *[R-101CC, 408655002] Status of intactness of mesorectal specimen (observable entity)*

*___ Not applicable *[R-101CD, 408656001] Intactness of mesorectal specimen not applicable (finding)*

*___ Complete *[R-101CE, 408657005] Mesorectal specimen completely intact (finding)*

*___ Near complete *[R-101CF, 408658000] Mesorectal specimen nearly completely intact (finding)*

*___ Incomplete *[R-101D0, 408659008] Intactness of mesorectal specimen incomplete (finding)*

Although the data item values remain the same (i.e., Not applicable, Complete), the associated SNOMED CT concepts and codes have changes. This illustrates the need for software systems using the CAP Cancer Checklists to monitor changes to the CAP Checklists and the SNOMED CT encoded Checklists and makes adjustments accordingly. Also, of note, during the course of this project the CAP Checklists went through considerable revisions to accommodate the new *American Joint Commission on Cancer, Tumor Node Metastases* (AJCC TNM), 6th edition, a clinical cancer staging schema.

During the course of this project, there was discussion about how much text as traditionally included in narrative style cancer pathology reports should be included along with the checklist data items. The findings indicate that some of the text information should remain. Clinical history is an example of useful cancer surveillance information that is typically included in narrative text and is not contained in the checklists. Other narrative text information could be useful within the cancer registry community. Allowing text in addition to the checklist data items could encourage pathologists to use the associated checklist software. Discussions with anatomical pathology LIS vendors indicate that this is the current strategy for product design.

Messaging

The process of obtaining consensus on the location of the information from the CAP checklists in the HL7 observation segment and the location of other header, patient, and physician identification information in the appropriate HL7 segments was time-consuming and challenging. The complexity of these issues is reflected in Appendix F, Message: Questions and Answers. During the course of this project, the NAACCR initiated a project to develop an HL7 message standard for the traditional narrative style pathology reports; a draft document has been posted (as of April 2005). This document addresses many of the same header, patient, and physician identification segments and will offer guidance to future implementers.

One concern raised during the Messaging Work Group meetings was the need for cancer registry software developers to be able to receive and process the checklists. As part of that process, the cancer registry software developers need to know which checklist is being received. Originally, the idea was to use the associated procedure code—i.e., "COLON AND RECTUM: Polypectomy P1-5700D Polypectomy - large intestine (procedure)." While this would work for the colon and rectum checklists, it would not have worked for other checklists, which could include multiple procedures—i.e., breast. As such the team asked for and received from the CAP Cancer Committee a "Checklist Identifier" concept code for each checklist. This concept will help software developers receiving electronic versions of this information to incorporate the data into the cancer registry software (and other) systems.

This concept created a unique challenge for the Messaging Work Group: where should this information be located in the HL7 message? After examining the possibility of using an OBX (Observation) segment, the work group agreed to use the OBR-44 (Observational request) procedure code segment for this information. Per the HL7 documentation, this segment "contains a unique identifier assigned to the procedure." Although not a procedure, this segment seemed the most appropriate and, as such, was used in this manner.

Related to this discussion was the issue of where to note in the HL7 message the SNOMED CT encoded CAP checklist version date. As noted in an earlier section, the SNOMED CT encoded CAP Cancer Checklists could change every January and July. The work group discussed the possibility of using the OBR-45 Procedure Code Modifier segment for this information. Another method discussed would be for the SNOMED CT CAP checklist encoders to change the checklist concept identification code with each version of the checklist. This would allow users to track version changes. Although these different options were discussed, no consensus was obtained and this remains an issue for future implementation.

The usual convention in the HL7 message is to use LOINC codes as the question codes and SNOMED CT codes for the answers. This project, to be consistent with national HL7 conventions and standards, used LOINC as the question codes and SNOMED CT codes for the answers. At the start of this project, LOINC codes did not exist for most of the CAP checklist question concepts. As such, during the course of this project, participants identified the colon and rectum cancer CAP checklist question concepts (or data items) and presented those concepts to the LOINC Clinical Committee for associated codes. Codes were subsequently issued for those concepts and used within the project messages. At the end of this project, LOINC codes do not exist for many of the non-colorectal cancer concepts. An examination of the SNOMED CT encoded checklists shows that SNOMED CT codes exist not only for the answer concepts but also for the question concepts. This raises the issue, within the context of the broader implementation of the CAP checklists, of whether the LOINC question concepts are necessary for implementation of the HL7 message of the SNOMED CT encoded CAP Cancer Checklists. This raises a related question about which codes are being used by software developers in the national community. While this project did not address that matter, the question is raised for future implementation.

Cancer Surveillance
One challenge facing the cancer surveillance community is identification of all cancers. There are multiple cancer case-finding sources, including disease indexes, but the primary source is pathology reports in anatomical pathology laboratories. More than 90% of all cancers were confirmed by positive microscopic findings (histology, cytology, or unspecified microscopy

method)[9]. Typically, a person trained in cancer identification rules visually scans each pathology and cytology report to identify a potential cancer. Within the realm of electronic pathology report cancer registration business rules (traditional narrative-text format), these digital reports are searched for key words and phrases to identify potential cancer reports. While implementation of the CAP cancer checklists can assist in the process of cancer identification, not all cancers will be identified. For example, in the Colon and Rectum Cancer Checklists, the protocol "applies to all invasive carcinomas of the colon and rectum. Carcinoid tumors, lymphomas, sarcomas, and tumors of the vermiform appendix are excluded" (Source: Appendix A). In addition, a checklist does not exist for incisional biopsy. Thus, cancer registries collecting the SNOMED CT encoded CAP checklist data will need to establish additional case-finding mechanisms to search and identify cancers from pathology reports using the traditional narrative-text format. Given these challenges, could systems be established within anatomical pathology laboratories to assist the cancer registration case-identification process?

Assessment
One of the project's limitations was the challenge of implementing a pilot project while running the routine system to process cancer pathology reports. This parallel process may have interfered with the assessment. In general, the participating pathologists did not process the cancer reports using the checklist data items until weeks or months after the initial reports had been processed. Consequently, entering the project cancers into the pilot systems may have become onerous and may have influenced pathologists' selection choices on the checklists. Retrospectively, pathologists should have been more active in the project activities.

As noted in the California and Ohio sections, both showed a loss of histology specificity, primarily in the area of adenocarcinoma in an adenoma. The number of histologies included in the CAP colorectal cancer checklist is limited to a choice of eight. Obviously, there are dozens of possible histologies for colorectal cancers. The idea behind the limited list is for pathologists to chose the "Other (specify)" option and then type in the more detailed histology. Apparently, participating pathologists rarely used the "Other (specify)" option. This could be due, in part, to the design of the pilot project, which involved a duplicate pathology report recording process. Perhaps the instructions on the SNOMED CT encoded CAP checklist and on the electronic versions, as developed by software vendors, need to be more explicit. From the cancer registry perspective this loss of histology specificity is a concern.

HISTOLOGIC TYPE
____ Adenocarcinoma
____ Mucinous adenocarcinoma (greater than 50% mucinous)
____ Medullary carcinoma
____ Signet-ring cell carcinoma (greater than 50% signet-ring cells)
____ Small cell carcinoma
____ Undifferentiated carcinoma
____ Other (specify): ____

---

[9] U.S. Cancer Statistics Working Group. *United States Cancer Statistics: 2001 Incidence and Mortality*. Atlanta (GA): Department of Health and Human Services, Centers for Disease Control and Prevention and National Caner Institute; 2004, p. 6

____ Carcinoma, type cannot be determined

In the Colon and Rectum: Polypectomy Checklist there is a concept related to "Type of polyp in which invasive carcinoma arose." This section was added in the January 2004 version of the checklist and is noted below. This information could have been used to code the more specific histologies for cancer registration for any polypectomy cases. In this project, Ohio had three polypectomy cases and California did not have any. This level of histology specificity is important for cancer surveillance and future implementations need to ensure that this information is captured in the cancer registry system. Possible solutions include use by pathologists of the "other (specify)" option or incorporating drop-down menus in the software, with listings of all possible histologies for the associated site. Site–histology tables are part of the cancer surveillance edits and include a list of all possible histologies by site. These tables are available at the National Cancer Institute Surveillance Epidemiology and End Results (NCI SEER) web site: http://seer.cancer.gov/icd-o-3/.

*TYPE OF POLYP IN WHICH INVASIVE CARCINOMA AROSE [R-101A8, 406126002] *Type of polyp from which malignant neoplasm originated (observable entity)* *___ Tubular [M-82110, 19665009] Tubular adenoma (morphologic abnormality)* *___ Villous [M-82610, 128859003] villous adenoma (morphologic abnormality)* *___ Tubulovillous [M-82630, 61722000] Tubulovillous adenoma (morphologic abnormality)* *___ Serrated [M-82130, 128653004] Serrated adenoma (morphologic abnormality)* *___ Hamartomatous [M-75660, 27391005] Hamartomatous polyp (morphologic abnormality)* *___ Indeterminate [R-100FA, 406012009] Polyp of indeterminate morphology (finding)*

Given these findings and the importance of histology data in cancer surveillance, it is interesting to examine the most common colorectal cancer histologies. The following table analyzes colon and rectum invasive cancers by the most frequently occurring histologies (the top 10). This table was produced from the United States Cancer Statistics, 2001 Incidence, database for colon and rectum cancers (including rectosigmoid) and excludes appendix, carcinoid tumors, sarcomas, and lymphomas for diagnosis year 2001. The histologies are sorted in descending order and show that "Adenocarcinoma, NOS" is the most commonly occurring histology for this site.

Of the seven histology choices [excluding "Other (specify)"] on the CAP colorectal cancer checklist, four are included in the table below: adenocarcinoma, NOS (81403) at approximately 70%; Mucinous adenocarcinoma (84803) at approximately 7%; Signet-ring cell carcinoma (84903) at approximately 1%; and Carcinoma, type cannot be determined (80103) at approximately <2%. The percentages of the remaining CAP colorectal cancer checklist histologies are as follows: small cell carcinoma (80413) at 0.09%, Undifferentiated carcinoma (80203) at 0.03%, and Medullary carcinoma (85103) at 0.01%.

Table 4
Colon and Rectum Cancers
Top Ten Histologies in Descending Order for Diagnosis Year 2001

Histology		2001		
Code	Name	Count	Column %	Cum %

81403	Adenocarcinoma, NOS	93,822	69.79	69.79
84803	Mucinous adenocarcinoma	9,507	7.07	76.86
82633	Adenocarcinoma in tubelovillous adenoma	7,720	5.74	82.60
82103	Adenocarcinoma in adenomatous polyp	6,229	4.63	87.23
82613	Adenocarcinoma in villous adenoma	3,898	2.90	90.13
84813	Mucin-producing adenocarcinoma	3,834	2.85	92.98
80003	Neoplasm, malignant	3,355	2.50	95.48
80103	Carcinoma, NOS	2,854	2.12	97.60
84903	Signet-ring cell carcinoma	1,385	1.03	98.63
80703	Squamous cell carcinoma, NOS	441	0.33	98.96

Note: Cum = cumulative, NOS = not otherwise specified.

As noted earlier two of the choices under Histologic Type include Mucinous adenocarcinoma and Signet-ring cell carcinoma, include some qualifiers: "Mucinous adenocarcinoma (greater than 50% mucinous)" and "Signet-ring cell carcinoma (greater than 50% signet-ring cells)." The corresponding guidance for cancer registrars is not as specific as the Checklist's "50%" criteria. There maybe a discrepancy between the coding rules used by pathologists and those used by cancer registrars.

The CAP Checklists, in addition to standard TNM codes, contain some additional codes: "pT3a/b" and "pT3c/d." These codes are not part of the AJCC TNM Manual, but they are part of the *TNM Supplement. A Commentary on Uniform Use*, 2nd edition, and are included in a chapter entitled "Optional Proposals for Testing New Telescopic Ramifications of TNM." Cancer registry software developers need to be aware of these obscure codes and convert accordingly.

While the checklists contained the items necessary to code the SEER Extent of Disease (EOD) stage data items, there was a loss of specificity in the Lymph Node data item. While regional lymph node involvement is included in the CAP cancer checklist, the location of the regional lymph node chain is not included. Below is a portion of the colon cancer SEER EOD table. Without the detailed lymph node chain information in the CAP checklists, 11 of the 50 cancers in the California assessment (22%) would have been coded to "3 – regional lymph nodes, NOS." Of note is that starting with cancers diagnosed on or after January 1, 2004, the SEER EOD staging schema was replaced with the *Collaborative Staging Manual and Coding Instructions*. This schema contains a "collaborative stage (CS) Lymph Nodes" data item that is nearly identical to the SEER EOD Lymph Node data item. This finding leads to several questions. What is the value of the specific regional lymph node chain for cancer surveillance? Why is this information included in the SEER EOD and CS Lymph Node data items but not in the CAP colon and rectum cancer checklist? Briefly, how significant is this loss of specificity?

REGIONAL Lymph Nodes

1 **All colon subsites:**
Epicolic (adjacent to bowel wall)
Paracolic/pericolic
Colic, NOS
Nodule(s) in pericolic fat

2 **Cecum and Appendix:**
Cecal: anterior, posterior, NOS
Ileocolic
Right colic

Ascending colon:
Ileocolic
Right colic
Middle colic

Transverse colon and flexures:
Middle colic
Right colic for **hepatic flexure only**
Left colic for **splenic flexure only**
Inferior mesenteric for **splenic flexure only**

Descending colon:
Left colic
Sigmoid
Inferior mesenteric

Sigmoid:
Sigmoidal (sigmoid mesenteric)
Superior hemorrhoidal
Superior rectal
Inferior mesenteric

3 Mesenteric, NOS
  Regional lymph node(s), NOS

Note: NOS = not otherwise specified.

Additional findings, observations, and conclusions about the California and Ohio assessments are included in the state-specific Challenges and Comments sections.

In the California assessment of the completeness rate for the required and not-required data elements identified for accreditation of cancer programs by the American College of Surgeons, CoC, of the 50 narrative reports, 20 reports (40%) were missing information for one or more of the checklist required data elements, and thus these checklist data elements could not be completed. Standard 4.6 of the American College of Surgeons, CoC Cancer Program Standards, 2004, states "The CoC requires that 90 percent of pathology reports that include a cancer diagnosis will contain the scientifically validated data elements outline on the surgical case summary checklist of the College of American Pathologists (CAP) publication, *Reporting on Cancer Specimens*." When this standard was applied to the 50 narrative reports reviewed, only 60% met the CoC standard.

Summary

The SNOMED CT encoded CAP Cancer Checklists offer significant opportunities and benefits for the cancer surveillance and anatomical pathology laboratory communities, although implementation challenges, as noted above, remain. Their use in hospital pathology laboratories that are part of a CoC approved cancer program can help to ensure that the associated CoC standard is met. Their use in the anatomical pathology laboratory with the appropriate software can form the basis of an anatomical pathology laboratory database, which has the potential to enhance clinical research and quality assurance studies. Their use in cancer registries can enhance existing systems and obviate much of the task of coding and entering data from the narrative text. The checklists could enhance the value to researchers who use the rapid case ascertainment systems of central cancer registries. In addition to obviating much of the task of coding, the checklists can make it possible to capture the intent of the pathologist at the point of diagnosis rather than the current method of cancer registrars interpreting text to derive the associated code. This allows for more accurate data collection by standardizing the meaning of the different concepts and the collection of more timely data by the electronic, real-time transmission to the cancer registry.

Appendices

Appendix A: College of American Pathologists Colon and Rectum Cancer Protocols and Checklists

- SNOMED CT Encoded – 2/04

Colon and Rectum

Protocol applies to all invasive carcinomas of the colon and rectum. Carcinoid tumors, lymphomas, sarcomas, and tumors of the vermiform appendix are excluded.

Protocol revision date: January 2004

Based on AJCC/UICC TNM, 6th edition

Procedures

- Incisional Biopsy (No Accompanying Checklist)
- Excisional Biopsy, Polypectomy
- Local Excision (Transanal Disk Excision)
- Segmental Resection
- Rectal Resection (Low Anterior Resection; Abdominoperineal Resection)

Author

Carolyn C. Compton, MD, PhD
        Department of Pathology, McGill University, Montreal, Quebec, Canada
For the Members of the Cancer Committee, College of American Pathologists

Previous contributors: Donald E. Henson, MD; Robert V.P. Hutter, MD; Leslie H. Sobin, MD; Harold E. Bowman, MD

The College of American Pathologists offers these protocols to assist pathologists in providing clinically useful and relevant information when reporting results of surgical specimen examinations of surgical specimens. The College regards the reporting elements in the "Surgical Pathology Cancer Case Summary (Checklist)" portion of the protocols as essential elements of the pathology report. However, the manner in which these elements are reported is at the discretion of each specific pathologist, taking into account clinician preferences, institutional policies, and individual practice.

The College developed these protocols as an educational tool to assist pathologists in the useful reporting of relevant information. It did not issue the protocols for use in litigation, reimbursement, or other contexts. Nevertheless, the College recognizes that the protocols might be used by hospitals, attorneys, payers, and others. Indeed, effective January 1, 2004, the Commission on Cancer of the American College of Surgeons mandated the use of the checklist elements of the protocols as part of its Cancer Program Standards for Approved Cancer Programs. Therefore, it becomes even more important for pathologists to familiarize themselves with the document. At the same time, the College cautions that use of the protocols other than for their intended educational purpose may involve additional considerations that are beyond the scope of this document

Summary of Changes to Checklist(s)

Protocol revision date: January 2004

The following changes have been made to the data elements of the checklist(s) since the January 2003 protocol revision.

Polypectomy Checklist

- Microscopic

- Margins: "Deep Margin" has been clarified as "Deep Margin (Stalk Margin)"
- Type of Polyp in Which Invasive Carcinoma Arose: this optional reporting element was added, as shown below

*Type of Polyp in Which Invasive Carcinoma Arose
   *___ Tubular
   *___ Villous
   *___ Tubulovillous
   *___ Serrated
   *___ Hamartomatous
   *___ Indeterminate

Colon and Rectum: Resection Checklist

Macroscopic

- Tumor Site: The reporting element "Colon, not otherwise specified" was added, as shown below

   Tumor site
   ___ Cecum
   ___ Right (ascending) colon
   ___ Hepatic flexure
   ___ Transverse colon
   ___ Splenic flexure
   ___ Left (descending) colon
   ___ Sigmoid colon
   ___ Rectosigmoid
   ___ Rectum

Appendix A: CAP Colon and Rectum Cancer Protocols and Checklists

___ Colon, not otherwise specified
___ Cannot be determined (see Comment)

- Margins: "Mesenteric Margin" was added as an optional reporting element, as shown below

*Mesenteric Margin
*___ Cannot be assessed
*___ Uninvolved by invasive carcinoma
*___ Involved by invasive carcinoma

Surgical Pathology Cancer Case Summary (Checklist)

Applies to invasive carcinomas only

Based on AJCC/UICC TNM, 6th edition

January 2004

Checklist identifier: [R-10117, 406031003] College of American Pathologists Cancer Checklist; Colon and Rectum: Polypectomy (qualifier value)

COLON AND RECTUM: Polypectomy *[P1-5700D, 235340004] Polypectomy - large intestine (procedure)*

[R-00254, 371439000] Specimen type (observable entity) and [G-8367, 122645001] Specimen from large intestine obtained by excisional biopsy (polypectomy) of lesion (specimen) these paired codes were added to capture specimen type implicit in checklist title.

Patient name: *[R-0025D, 371484003] Patient name (observable entity)*
Surgical pathology number: *[R-002A2, 371482004] Surgical pathology identifier (observable entity)*

Note: Check 1 response unless otherwise indicated.

MACROSCOPIC *[F-048D6, 395526000] Macroscopic specimen observable (observable entity)*

TUMOR SITE *[R-0025A, 371480007] Tumor site (observable entity)*
___ Cecum *[T-59100, 32713005] Cecum structure (body structure)*
___ Right (ascending) colon *[T-59400, 51342009] Right colon structure (body structure)*
___ Hepatic flexure *[T-59438, 48338005] Structure of right colic flexure (body structure)*
___ Transverse colon *[T-59440, 485005] Transverse colon structure (body structure)*
___ Splenic flexure *[T-59442, 72592005] Structure of left colic flexure (body structure)*
___ Left (descending) colon *[T-59450, 55572008] Left colon structure (body structure)*
___ Sigmoid colon *[T-59470, 60184004] Sigmoid colon structure (body structure)*

___ Rectum *[T-59600, 34402009] Rectum structure (body structure)*
___ Not specified *[T-59000, 14742008] Large intestinal structure (body structure)*

POLYP SIZE *[R-00294, 372258008] Polyp size (observable entity)*
Greatest dimension: ___ cm *[R-00286, 373197004] Polyp size, largest dimension (observable entity)*
*Additional dimensions: ___ x ___ cm *[R-0045A, 395509006] Polyp size, additional dimension (observable entity)*
___ Cannot be determined (see Comment) *[R-100A5, 397361006] Polyp size cannot be determined (finding)*

POLYP CONFIGURATION *[R-002AC, 371501006] Polyp configuration (observable entity)*
___ Pedunculated with stalk *[R-1005C, 395498009] Pedunculated polyp with stalk (morphologic abnormality)*
   Stalk length: ___ cm *[R-0045B, 395511002] Polyp stalk length (observable entity)*
___ Pedunculated, no stalk *[R-1005D, 395499001] Pedunculated polyp without stalk (morphologic abnormality)*
___ Sessile *[M-76801, 103679000] Sessile polyp (morphologic abnormality)*
___ Fragmented *[F-02BAB, 395528004] Tissue specimen fragmented (finding)*

MICROSCOPIC *[F-048D7, 395527009] Microscopic specimen observable (observable entity)*

HISTOLOGIC TYPE *[R-00257, 371441004] Histologic type (observable entity)*
___ Adenocarcinoma *[M-81403, 35917007] Adenocarcinoma, no subtype (morphologic abnormality)*
___ Mucinous adenocarcinoma (greater than 50% mucinous) *[M-84803, 72495009] Mucinous adenocarcinoma (morphologic abnormality)*
___ Medullary carcinoma *[M-85103, 32913002] Medullary carcinoma (morphologic abnormality)*
___ Signet-ring cell carcinoma (greater than 50% signet-ring cells) *[M-84903, 87737001] Signet ring cell carcinoma (morphologic abnormality)*
___ Small cell carcinoma *[M-80413, 74364000] Small cell carcinoma (morphologic abnormality)*
___ Undifferentiated carcinoma *[M-80203, 38549000] Carcinoma, undifferentiated (morphologic abnormality)*
___ Other (specify): ___ *not coded*
___ Carcinoma, type cannot be determined *[M-80103, 68453008] Carcinoma, no subtype (morphologic abnormality)*

HISTOLOGIC GRADE *[R-00258, 371469007] Histologic grade (observable entity)*
___ Not applicable *[G-F505, 60815008] Grade not determined (finding)*
___ Cannot be determined *[R-00436, 384741006] Grade cannot be determined (finding)*
___ Low-grade (well or moderately differentiated) *[F-02BAC, 395529007] Low grade (well to moderately differentiated) (finding)*
___ High-grade (poorly differentiated to undifferentiated) *[F-02BAD, 395530002] High grade (poorly differentiated to undifferentiated) (finding)*

Appendix A: CAP Colon and Rectum Cancer Protocols and Checklists

EXTENT OF INVASION *[R-00259, 371487005] Tumor extent of invasion (observable entity)*
___ Cannot be determined *[F-02BAE, 395532005] Tumor extent of invasion cannot be determined (finding)*
Invasion (deepest): *not coded*
___ Lamina propria *[R-0046E, 395533000] Tumor invades lamina propria (finding)*
___ Muscularis mucosae *[R-0046F, 395534006] Tumor invades muscularis mucosae (finding)*
___ Submucosa *[G-F7AB, 370059003] Tumor invasion into submucosa (finding)*
___ Muscularis propria *[G-F7AC, 370060008] Tumor invasion into muscularis propria (finding)*

MARGINS (check all that apply) *[R-100D3, 399677006] Status of surgical margin involvement by tumor in polypectomy specimen (observable entity)*

Deep margin (Stalk margin) *[R-00479, 395543002] Status of surgical deep margin involvement by tumor (observable entity) this concept will need to be combined with concept above*
___ Cannot be assessed *[R-0055D, 399652005] Surgical deep margin involvement by tumor cannot be assessed (finding)*
___ Uninvolved by invasive carcinoma *[R-0047D, 395547001] surgical deep margin uninvolved by malignant neoplasm (finding)*
    Distance of invasive carcinoma from margin: ___ mm *[R-00468, 385390003] Distance of malignant neoplasm from deep margin (observable entity)*
___ Involved by invasive carcinoma *[R-0047A, 395544008] surgical deep margin involved by malignant neoplasm (finding)*

Mucosal/Lateral margin *[R-00437, 384786009] Status of surgical lateral (mucosal/mural) margin involvement by tumor (observable entity)*
___ Not applicable *[R-100A6, 397362004] surgical lateral (mucosal/mural) margin involvement by tumor not applicable (finding)*
___ Cannot be assessed *[R-100F9, 405980004] Surgical lateral (mucosal/mural) margin involvement by tumor cannot be assessed (finding)*
___ Uninvolved by invasive carcinoma *[R-0045E, 384804002] surgical lateral (mucosal/mural) margin uninvolved by malignant neoplasm (finding)*
___ Involved by invasive carcinoma *[R-0045C, 384801005] surgical lateral (mucosal/mural) margin involved by malignant neoplasm (finding)*
___ Involved by in situ carcinoma/adenoma *[R-100AA, 397189000] surgical lateral (mucosal/mural) margin involved by in situ carcinoma/adenoma (finding)*

LYMPHATIC (SMALL VESSEL) INVASION (L) *[R-00404, 395715009] Status of lymphatic (small vessel) invasion by tumor (observable entity)*
___ Absent *[G-F220, 44649003] L0 stage (finding)*
___ Present *[G-F221, 74139005] L1 stage (finding)*
___ Indeterminate *[G-F225, 33419001] LX stage (finding)*

*VENOUS (LARGE VESSEL) INVASION (V) *[R-00270, 371493002] Status of venous (large vessel) invasion by tumor (observable entity)*
*___ Absent *[G-F230, 40223008] V0 stage (finding)*
*___ Present *[G-F539, 369732007] Venous (large vessel) invasion by tumor present (finding)*

*___ Indeterminate *[G-F235, 6510002] VX stage (finding)*

*TYPE OF POLYP IN WHICH INVASIVE CARCINOMA AROSE *[R-101A8, 406126002]*
Type of polyp from which malignant neoplasm originated (observable entity)
*___ Tubular *[M-82110, 19665009] Tubular adenoma (morphologic abnormality)*
*___ Villous *[M-82610, 128859003] villous adenoma (morphologic abnormality)*
*___ Tubulovillous *[M-82630, 61722000] Tubulovillous adenoma (morphologic abnormality)*
*___ Serrated *[M-82130, 128653004] Serrated adenoma (morphologic abnormality)*
*___ Hamartomatous *[M-75660, 27391005] Hamartomatous polyp (morphologic abnormality)*
*___ Indeterminate *[R-100FA, 406012009] Polyp of indeterminate morphology (finding)*

*ADDITIONAL PATHOLOGIC FINDINGS (check all that apply) *[R-0025E, 371498006]*
   Additional pathologic finding in tumor specimen (observable entity)
*___ None identified *[F-02BB1, 395555008] No additional pathologic finding in tumor*
   specimen (finding)
*___ Active colitis *[D5-41700, 64226004] Colitis (disorder)*
*___ Other (specify):___ *not coded*

*COMMENT(S)

Surgical Pathology Cancer Case Summary (Checklist)

Applies to invasive carcinomas only

Based on AJCC/UICC TNM, 6th edition

January 2004

Checklist identifier: [R-10118, 406032005] College of American Pathologists Cancer Checklist;
Rectum: Local Excision (Transanal Disk Excision) (qualifier value)
RECTUM: Local Excision (Transanal Disk Excision) *[P1-5832A, 287784004] Local excision*
of rectum (procedure)

[R-00254, 371439000] Specimen type (observable entity) and [G-8376, 122653009] Specimen
from rectum obtained by transanal disk excision (specimen) these paired codes were added to
capture the specimen type implicit in the checklist title.

Patient name: *[R-0025D, 371484003] Patient name (observable entity)*
Surgical pathology number: *[R-002A2, 371482004] Surgical pathology identifier (observable*
entity)

Note: Check 1 response unless otherwise indicated.

MACROSCOPIC *[F-048D6, 395526000] Macroscopic specimen observable (observable entity)*

SPECIMEN INTEGRITY *[R-100A8, 397191008] Specimen integrity (observable entity)*
___ Intact *[R-100A9, 397315006] Tissue specimen intact (finding)*
___ Fragmented *[F-02BAB, 395528004] Tissue specimen fragmented (finding)*
 *Number of pieces: ___ *[F-048D8, 395558005] Number of pieces in fragmented specimen (observable entity)*

*TUMOR SITE *[R-0025A, 371480007] Tumor site (observable entity) and [T-59600, 34402009] Rectum structure (body structure) Will require two codes to capture tumor site implied in checklist title*
*Distance from anal verge (per clinical report): ___ cm *[R-00266, 371490004] Distance of tumor from anal verge (observable entity)*
*___ Distance from anal verge unknown *[R-0027C, 372298005] Distance of tumor from anal verge unknown (finding) this answers [R-00266, 371490004] Distance of tumor from anal verge (observable entity)*

*TUMOR CONFIGURATION *[R-002AD, 371500007] Tumor configuration (observable entity)*
*___ Exophytic (polypoid) *[G-F576, 369749000] Exophytic (polypoid) tumor configuration (finding)*
*___ Infiltrative *[G-F579, 369752008] Infiltrative tumor configuration, macroscopic (finding)*
*___ Ulcerating *[G-F57D, 369760009] Ulcerated tumor configuration (finding)*
*___ Other (specify): ___ *not coded*

TUMOR SIZE *[F-02BBE, 263605001] Tumor size (observable entity)*
Greatest dimension: ___ cm *[R-00272, 371479009] Tumor size, largest dimension (observable entity)*
*Additional dimensions: ___ x ___ cm *[F-02BDC, 395512009] Tumor size, additional dimension (observable entity)*
___ Cannot be determined (see Comment) *[R-100A7, 396919000] Tumor size cannot be assessed (finding)*

MICROSCOPIC *[F-048D7, 395527009] Microscopic specimen observable (observable entity)*

HISTOLOGIC TYPE *[R-00257, 371441004] Histologic type (observable entity)*
___ Adenocarcinoma *[M-81403, 35917007] Adenocarcinoma, no subtype (morphologic abnormality)*
___ Mucinous adenocarcinoma (greater than 50% mucinous) *[M-84803, 72495009] Mucinous adenocarcinoma (morphologic abnormality)*
___ Medullary carcinoma *[M-85103, 32913002] medullary carcinoma (morphologic abnormality)*
___ Signet-ring cell carcinoma (greater than 50% signet-ring cells) *[M-84903, 87737001] Signet ring cell carcinoma (morphologic abnormality)*

___ Small cell carcinoma *[M-80413, 74364000] Small cell carcinoma (morphologic abnormality)*

___ Undifferentiated carcinoma *[M-80203, 38549000] Carcinoma, undifferentiated (morphologic abnormality)*

___ Other (specify): ___ *not coded*

___ Carcinoma, type cannot be determined *[M-80103, 68453008] Carcinoma, no subtype (morphologic abnormality)*

HISTOLOGIC GRADE *[R-00258, 371469007] Histologic grade (observable entity)*

___ Not applicable *[G-F505, 60815008] Grade not determined (finding)*

___ Cannot be assessed *[R-00436, 384741006] Grade cannot be determined (finding)*

___ Low-grade (well or moderately differentiated) *[F-02BAC, 395529007] Low grade (well to moderately differentiated) (finding)*

___ High-grade (poorly differentiated to undifferentiated) *[F-02BAD, 395530002] High grade (poorly differentiated to undifferentiated) (finding)*

PATHOLOGIC STAGING (pTNM) *[R-100F7, 405979002] Pathologic TNM stage (observable entity)*

PRIMARY TUMOR (pT) *[R-00415, 384625004] pT category (observable entity)*

___ pTX: Cannot be assessed *[G-F187, 43189003] pTX category (finding)*

___ pT0:   No evidence of primary tumor *[G-F182, 39880006] pT0 category (finding)*

___ pTis: Carcinoma in situ, intraepithelial (no invasion) *[G-F196, 395705003] pTis: Carcinoma in situ, intraepithelial (colon/rectum) (finding)*

___ pTis: Carcinoma in situ, invasion of lamina propria *[G-F73E, 373201004] pTis: Carcinoma in situ, invasion of lamina propria (finding)*

___ pT1:   Tumor invades submucosa *[G-F6A0, 373200003] pT1: Tumor invades submucosa (colon/rectum) (finding)*

___ pT2:   Tumor invades muscularis propria *[G-F197, 395706002] pT2: Tumor invades muscularis propria (colon/rectum) (finding)*

___ pT3:   Tumor invades through the muscularis propria into the subserosa or the nonperitonealized pericolic or perirectal soft tissues *[G-F198, 395707006] pT3: Tumor invades through the muscularis propria into the subserosa or into non-peritonealized pericolic or perirectal tissues (colon/rectum) (finding)*

*____ pT3a/b: Tumor invades through the muscularis propria into the subserosa or the nonperitonealized pericolic or perirectal soft   tissues, invades 5 mm or less beyond the border of the muscularis propria *[G-F199, 395708001] pT3a,b: Tumor invades through the muscularis propria into the subserosa or into non-peritonealized pericolic or perirectal tissues, invades 5 mm or less beyond the border of the muscularis propria (colon/rectum) (finding)*

*____ pT3c/d: Tumor invades through the muscularis propria into the subserosa or the nonperitonealized pericolic or perirectal soft tissues, invades greater than 5 mm beyond the border of the muscularis propria *[G-F19A, 395709009] pT3c, d: Tumor invades through the muscularis propria into the subserosa or into non-peritonealized pericolic or perirectal tissues, invades greater than 5 mm beyond the border of the muscularis propria (colon/rectum) (finding)*

Appendix A: CAP Colon and Rectum Cancer Protocols and Checklists

___ pT4:   Tumor directly invades adjacent structures *[G-F19B, 395710004] pT4: Tumor directly invades other organs or structures and/or perforates visceral peritoneum (colon/rectum) (finding)*

REGIONAL LYMPH NODES (pN) *[R-0026B, 371494008] pN category (observable entity)*
___ pNX: Cannot be assessed *[G-F195, 54452005] pNX category (finding)*
___ pN0: No regional lymph node metastasis *[G-F190, 21917009] pN0 category (finding)*
___ pN1: Metastasis in 1 to 3 lymph nodes *[G-F19C, 395711000] pN1: Metastasis in 1 to 3 regional lymph nodes (colon/rectum) (finding)*
___ pN2: Metastasis in 4 or more lymph nodes *[G-F19D, 395712007] pN2: Metastasis in 4 or more regional lymph nodes (colon/rectum) (finding)*
Specify: Number examined: ___ *[R-002AA, 372309006] Number of regional lymph nodes examined (observable entity)*
             Number involved: ___ *[R-002AB, 372308003] Number of regional lymph nodes involved (observable entity)*

MARGINS (check all that apply) *[R-00472, 395535007] Status of surgical margin involvement by tumor (observable entity)*

Lateral Margin *[R-00437, 384786009] Status of surgical lateral (mucosal/mural) margin involvement by tumor (observable entity)*
___ Cannot be assessed *[R-100F9, 405980004] Surgical lateral (mucosal/mural) margin involvement by tumor cannot be assessed (finding)*
___ Uninvolved by invasive carcinoma *[R-0045E, 384804002] surgical lateral (mucosal/mural) margin uninvolved by malignant neoplasm (finding)*
      Distance of invasive carcinoma from closest lateral margin: ___ mm
      [R-0046B, 385393001] Distance of malignant neoplasm from closest lateral margin (observable entity)
          Specify location (eg, o'clock position), if possible: ____ not coded
___ Involved by invasive carcinoma *[R-0045C, 384801005] surgical lateral (mucosal/mural) margin involved by malignant neoplasm (finding)*
          Specify location (eg, o'clock position), if possible: ____ not coded
*___ Involved by carcinoma in situ/adenoma *[R-100AA, 397189000] Surgical lateral (mucosal/mural) margin involved by in situ carcinoma/adenoma (finding)*

Deep Margin *[R-00479, 395543002] Status of surgical deep margin involvement by tumor (observable entity)*
___ Cannot be assessed *[R-0055D, 399652005] Surgical deep margin involvement by tumor cannot be assessed (finding)*
___ Uninvolved by invasive carcinoma *[R-0047D, 395547001] surgical deep margin uninvolved by malignant neoplasm (finding)*
      Distance of invasive carcinoma from margin: ___ mm *[R-00468, 385390003] Distance of malignant neoplasm from deep margin (observable entity)*
___ Focal involvement by invasive carcinoma *[R-00402, 395713002] Surgical deep margin involved by malignant neoplasm, focal (finding)*
___ Multifocal involvement by invasive carcinoma *[R-00403, 395714008] Surgical deep margin involved by malignant neoplasm, multifocal (finding)*

Appendix A: CAP Colon and Rectum Cancer Protocols and Checklists

LYMPHATIC (SMALL VESSEL) INVASION (L) (check all that apply) *[R-00404, 395715009]*
     Status of lymphatic (small vessel) invasion by tumor (observable entity)
___ Absent *[G-F220, 44649003] L0 stage (finding)*
___ Present *[G-F221, 74139005] L1 stage (finding)*
          *___ Intramural *[F-02B82, 395718006] Lymphatic (small vessel) intramural invasion by
     tumor present (finding)*
               *___ Extramural *[F-02B83, 395719003] Lymphatic (small vessel) extramural invasion
               by tumor present (finding)*
___ Indeterminate *[G-F225, 33419001] LX stage (finding)*

VENOUS (LARGE VESSEL) INVASION (V) (check all that apply) *[R-00270, 371493002]*
     Status of venous (large vessel) invasion by tumor (observable entity)
___ Absent *[G-F230, 40223008] V0 stage (finding)*
___ Present *[G-F539, 369732007] Venous (large vessel) invasion by tumor present (finding)*
               *___ Intramural *[G-F53A, 369733002] Venous (large vessel) intramural invasion by
               tumor present (finding)*
               *___ Extramural *[G-F53B, 369734008] Venous (large vessel) extramural invasion by
               tumor present (finding)*
___ Indeterminate *[G-F235, 6510002] VX stage (finding)*

*PERINEURAL INVASION *[R-0026D, 371513001] Status of perineural invasion by tumor
     (observable entity)*
* ___ Absent *[G-F7A3, 370051000] Perineural invasion by tumor absent (finding)*
* ___ Present *[G-F538, 369731000] Perineural invasion by tumor present (finding)*

*TUMOR BORDER CONFIGURATION *[R-00260, 371502004] Tumor border configuration
     (observable entity)*
* ___ Pushing *[G-F562, 369742009] Pushing tumor border (finding)*
* ___ Infiltrating *[G-F561, 369741002] Infiltrating tumor border, microscopic (finding)*

*INTRATUMORAL/PERITUMORAL LYMPHOCYTIC RESPONSE *[R-00407, 384604004]
     Status of intratumoral/peritumoral lymphocyte response (observable entity)*
* ___ None *[F-D0193, 384601007] Intratumoral/peritumoral lymphocytic response absent
     (finding)*
* ___ Mild to moderate *[F-D0194, 384602000] Intratumoral/peritumoral lymphocytic response
     mild to moderate (finding)*
* ___ Marked (including Crohn-like response) *[R-00406, 384603005] Intratumoral/peritumoral
lymphocytic response marked (finding)*

*ADDITIONAL PATHOLOGIC FINDINGS (check all that apply) *[R-0025E, 371498006]*
     Additional pathologic finding in tumor specimen (observable entity)
* ___ None identified *[F-02BB1, 395555008] No additional pathologic finding in tumor
     specimen (finding)*
* ___ Adenoma(s) *[R-100D4, 399730005] Adenoma of rectum (disorder)*
* ___ Chronic ulcerative proctocolitis *[D5-45281, 295046003] Ulcerative proctocolitis
     (disorder)*

*___ Crohn disease *[D5-41000, 34000006] Crohn's disease (disorder)*
*___ Dysplasia *[D5-40049, 308875009] Dysplasia of rectum (disorder)*
*___ Other polyps (type[s]):___ *[D5-45320, 39772007] rectal polyp (disorder)*
*___ Other (specify): ___ *not coded*

*COMMENT(S)

Surgical Pathology Cancer Case Summary (Checklist)

Applies to invasive carcinomas only

Based on AJCC/UICC TNM, 6th edition

January 2004

Checklist identifier: [R-10119, 406033000] College of American Pathologists Cancer Checklist; Colon and Rectum: Resection (qualifier value)
COLON AND RECTUM: Resection *[P1-573F9, 107944001] Large intestine excision (procedure)*

Patient name: *[R-0025D, 371484003] Patient name (observable entity)*
Surgical pathology number: *[R-002A2, 371482004] Surgical pathology identifier (observable entity)*
Other identifiers: *not coded*

Note: Check 1 response unless otherwise indicated.

MACROSCOPIC *[F-048D6, 395526000] Macroscopic specimen observable (observable entity)*

SPECIMEN TYPE *[R-00254, 371439000] Specimen type (observable entity)*
___ Right hemicolectomy *[G-8371, 122648004] Specimen from colon obtained by right hemicolectomy (specimen)*
   *Length: ___ cm *[R-00408, 384606002] Length of specimen (observable entity)*
___ Transverse colectomy *[G-8372, 122649007] Specimen from colon obtained by transverse colectomy (specimen)*
   *Length: ___ cm *[R-00408, 384606002] Length of specimen (observable entity)*
___ Left hemicolectomy *[G-8373, 122650007] Specimen from colon obtained by left hemicolectomy (specimen)*
   *Length: ___ cm *[R-00408, 384606002] Length of specimen (observable entity)*
___ Sigmoidectomy *[G-8374, 122651006] Specimen from colon obtained by sigmoidectomy (specimen)*
   *Length: ___ cm *[R-00408, 384606002] Length of specimen (observable entity)*

___ Rectal/rectosigmoid colon (low anterior resection) *[G-8375, 122652004] Specimen from colon obtained by rectal/rectosigmoid (low anterior) resection (specimen)*
     Length: ___ cm [R-00408, 384606002] Length of specimen (observable entity)
___ Total abdominal colectomy *[G-8369, 122647009] Specimen from large intestine obtained by total abdominal colectomy (specimen)*
     Length: ___ cm [R-00408, 384606002] Length of specimen (observable entity)
___ Abdominoperineal resection *[G-8368, 122646000] Specimen from large intestine obtained by abdominoperineal resection (specimen)*
     Length: ___ cm [R-00408, 384606002] Length of specimen (observable entity)
___ Other (specify): ___ *not coded*
     Length: ___ cm [R-00408, 384606002] Length of specimen (observable entity)
___ Not specified *[G-8365, 122643008] Tissue specimen from large intestine (specimen)*

TUMOR SITE *[R-0025A, 371480007] Tumor site (observable entity)*
___ Cecum *[T-59100, 32713005] Cecum structure (body structure)*
___ Right (ascending) colon *[T-59400, 51342009] Right colon structure (body structure)*
___ Hepatic flexure *[T-59438, 48338005] Structure of right colic flexure (body structure)*
___ Transverse colon *[T-59440, 485005] Transverse colon structure (body structure)*
___ Splenic flexure *[T-59442, 72592005] Structure of left colic flexure (body structure)*
___ Left (descending) colon *[T-59450, 55572008] Left colon structure (body structure)*
___ Sigmoid colon *[T-59470, 60184004] Sigmoid colon structure (body structure)*
___ Rectosigmoid *[T-59680, 81922002] Rectosigmoid structure (body structure)*
___ Rectum *[T-59600, 34402009] Rectum structure (body structure)*
___ Colon, not otherwise specified *[T-59300, 71854001] Colon structure (body structure)*
___ Cannot be determined (see Comment) *[T-59000, 14742008] Large intestinal structure (body structure)*

*TUMOR CONFIGURATION *[R-002AD, 371500007] Tumor configuration (observable entity)*
*___ Exophytic (polypoid) *[G-F576, 369749000] Exophytic (polypoid) tumor configuration (finding)*
*___ Infiltrative *[G-F579, 369752008] Infiltrative tumor configuration, macroscopic (finding)*
*___ Ulcerating *[G-F57D, 369760009] Ulcerated tumor configuration (finding)*
*___ Other (specify): __*not coded*

TUMOR SIZE *[F-02BBE, 263605001] Tumor size (observable entity)*
Greatest dimension: ___ cm *[R-00272, 371479009] Tumor size, largest dimension (observable entity)*
*Additional dimensions: ___ x ___ cm *[F-02BDC, 395512009] Tumor size, additional dimension (observable entity)*
___ Cannot be determined (see Comment) *[R-100A7, 396919000] Tumor size cannot be assessed (finding)*

*MESORECTUM *[G-F7B9, 384607006] Status of invasion of mesorectum by tumor (observable entity)*
*___ Not applicable *[F-02B8F, 384611000] Invasion of mesorectum by tumor not applicable (finding)*
*___ Complete *[R-00409, 384608001] complete invasion of mesorectum by tumor (finding)*

Appendix A: CAP Colon and Rectum Cancer Protocols and Checklists

*___ Near complete *[R-0040A, 384609009] Near complete invasion of mesorectum by tumor (finding)*
*___ Incomplete *[R-0040B, 384610004] incomplete invasion of mesorectum by tumor (finding)*

MICROSCOPIC *[F-048D7, 395527009] Microscopic specimen observable (observable entity)*

HISTOLOGIC TYPE *[R-00257, 371441004] Histologic type (observable entity)*
___ Adenocarcinoma *[M-81403, 35917007] Adenocarcinoma, no subtype (morphologic abnormality)*
___ Mucinous adenocarcinoma (greater than 50% mucinous) *[M-84803, 72495009] Mucinous adenocarcinoma (morphologic abnormality)*
___ Medullary carcinoma *[M-85103, 32913002] Medullary carcinoma (morphologic abnormality)*
___ Signet-ring cell carcinoma (greater than 50% signet-ring cells) *[M-84903, 87737001] Signet ring cell carcinoma (morphologic abnormality)*
___ Small cell carcinoma *[M-80413, 74364000] Small cell carcinoma (morphologic abnormality)*
___ Undifferentiated carcinoma *[M-80203, 38549000] Carcinoma, undifferentiated (morphologic abnormality)*
___ Other (specify): __ *not coded*
___ Carcinoma, type cannot be determined *[M-80103, 68453008] Carcinoma, no subtype (morphologic abnormality)*

HISTOLOGIC GRADE *[R-00258, 371469007] Histologic grade (observable entity)*
___ Not applicable *[G-F505, 60815008] Grade not determined (finding)*
___ Cannot be assessed *[R-00436, 384741006] Grade cannot be determined (finding)*
___ Low-grade (well or moderately differentiated) *[F-02BAC, 395529007] Low grade (well to moderately differentiated) (finding)*
___ High-grade (poorly differentiated to undifferentiated) *[F-02BAD, 395530002] High grade (poorly differentiated to undifferentiated) (finding)*
___ Other (specify): ____*not coded*

PATHOLOGIC STAGING (pTNM) *[R-100F7, 405979002] Pathologic TNM stage (observable entity)*

PRIMARY TUMOR (pT) *[R-00415, 384625004] pT category (observable entity)*
___ pTX: Cannot be assessed *[G-F187, 43189003] pTX category (finding)*
___ pT0:   No evidence of primary tumor *[G-F182, 39880006] pT0 category (finding)*
___ pTis: Carcinoma in situ, intraepithelial (no invasion) *[G-F196, 395705003] pTis: Carcinoma in situ, intraepithelial (colon/rectum) (finding)*
___ pTis: Carcinoma in situ, invasion of lamina propria *[G-F73E, 373201004] pTis: Carcinoma in situ, invasion of lamina propria (finding)*
___ pT1:   Tumor invades submucosa *[G-F6A0, 373200003] pT1: Tumor invades submucosa (colon/rectum) (finding)*
___ pT2:   Tumor invades muscularis propria *[G-F197, 395706002] pT2: Tumor invades muscularis propria (colon/rectum) (finding)*

Appendix A: CAP Colon and Rectum Cancer Protocols and Checklists

___ pT3:   Tumor invades through the muscularis propria into the subserosa or the nonperitonealized pericolic or perirectal soft tissues *[G-F198, 395707006] pT3: Tumor invades through the muscularis propria into the subserosa or into non-peritonealized pericolic or perirectal tissues (colon/rectum) (finding)*

*___ pT3a/b: Tumor invades through the muscularis propria into the subserosa or the nonperitonealized pericolic or perirectal soft   tissues, invades 5 mm or less beyond the border of the muscularis propria *[G-F199, 395708001] pT3a,b: Tumor invades through the muscularis propria into the subserosa or into non-peritonealized pericolic or perirectal tissues, invades 5 mm or less beyond the border of the muscularis propria (colon/rectum) (finding)*

*___ pT3c/d: Tumor invades through the muscularis propria into the subserosa or the nonperitonealized pericolic or perirectal soft tissues, invades greater than 5 mm beyond the border of the muscularis propria *[G-F19A, 395709009] pT3c, d: Tumor invades through the muscularis propria into the subserosa or into non-peritonealized pericolic or perirectal tissues, invades greater than 5 mm beyond the border of the muscularis propria (colon/rectum) (finding)*

___ pT4a: Tumor directly invades other organs or structures *[G-F19E, 384612007] pT4a: Tumor directly invades other organs or structures (colon/rectum) (finding)*

___ pT4b: Tumor penetrates the visceral peritoneum *[G-F19F, 384613002] pT4b: Tumor penetrates visceral peritoneum (colon/rectum) (finding)*

REGIONAL LYMPH NODES (pN) *[R-0026B, 371494008] pN category (observable entity)*
___ pNX: Cannot be assessed *[G-F195, 54452005] pNX category (finding)*
___ pN0: No regional lymph node metastasis *[G-F190, 21917009] pN0 category (finding)*
___ pN1: Metastasis in 1 to 3 regional lymph nodes *[G-F19C, 395711000] pN1: Metastasis in 1 to 3 regional lymph nodes (colon/rectum) (finding)*
___ pN2: Metastasis in 4 or more regional lymph nodes *[G-F19D, 395712007] pN2: Metastasis in 4 or more regional lymph nodes (colon/rectum) (finding)*
Specify: Number examined: ___ *[R-002AA, 372309006] Number of regional lymph nodes examined (observable entity)*
Number involved: ___ *[R-002AB, 372308003] Number of regional lymph nodes involved (observable entity)*

DISTANT METASTASIS (pM) *[R-00269, 371497001] pM category (observable entity)*
___ pMX: Cannot be assessed *[G-F205, 17076002] pMX stage (finding)*
___ pM1: Distant metastasis *[G-F201, 14926007] pM1 stage (finding)*
*Specify site(s):___ *[R-10063, 385421009] Site of distant metastasis (observable entity)*

MARGINS (check all that apply) *[R-00472, 395535007] Status of surgical margin involvement by tumor (observable entity)*

Proximal Margin *[R-002B6, 372439002] Status of surgical proximal margin involvement by tumor (observable entity)*
___Cannot be assessed *[R-00570, 399609005] Surgical proximal margin involvement by tumor cannot be assessed (finding)*

___ Uninvolved by invasive carcinoma *[R-0040C, 384614008] surgical proximal margin uninvolved by malignant neoplasm (finding)*
___ Involved by invasive carcinoma *[R-0040D, 384615009] surgical proximal margin involved by malignant neoplasm (finding)*
___ Carcinoma in situ/adenoma absent at proximal margin *[R-0041A, 384637002] surgical proximal margin uninvolved by in situ carcinoma/adenoma (finding)*
___ Carcinoma in situ/adenoma present at proximal margin *[R-0041B, 384638007] surgical proximal margin involved by in situ carcinoma/adenoma (finding)*

Distal Margin *[R-002B5, 372440000] Status of surgical distal margin involvement by tumor (observable entity)*
___Cannot be assessed *[R-00507, 399555002] Surgical distal margin involvement by tumor cannot be assessed (finding)*
___ Uninvolved by invasive carcinoma *[R-00414, 384623006] surgical distal margin uninvolved by malignant neoplasm (finding)*
___ Involved by invasive carcinoma *[G-8DA7, 384622001] surgical distal margin involved by malignant neoplasm (finding)*
___ Carcinoma in situ/adenoma absent at distal margin *[R-0041D, 384640002] surgical distal margin uninvolved by in situ carcinoma/adenoma (finding)*
___ Carcinoma in situ/adenoma present at distal margin *[R-0041C, 384639004] surgical distal margin involved by in situ carcinoma/adenoma (finding)*

Circumferential (Radial) Margin *[R-00410, 384618006] Status of surgical circumferential margin involvement by tumor (observable entity)*
___ Not applicable *[R-00411, 384619003] Surgical circumferential margin involvement by tumor not applicable (finding)*
___Cannot be assessed *[R-00573, 399664002] Surgical circumferential margin involvement by tumor cannot be assessed (finding)*
___ Uninvolved by invasive carcinoma *[R-00413, 384621008] surgical circumferential margin uninvolved by malignant neoplasm (finding)*
___ Involved by invasive carcinoma (tumor present 0-1 mm from CRM) *[R-00412, 384620009] Surgical circumferential margin involved by malignant neoplasm (tumor present 0-1 mm from CRM) (finding)*

*Mesenteric Margin *[R-100FD, 405981000] Status of surgical mesenteric margin involvement by tumor (observable entity)*
*___ Cannot be assessed *[R-100FE, 405982007] Surgical mesenteric margin involvement by tumor cannot be assessed (finding)*
*___ Uninvolved by invasive carcinoma *[R-100FF, 405984008] surgical mesenteric margin uninvolved by malignant neoplasm (finding)*
*___ Involved by invasive carcinoma *[R-10100, 405985009] surgical mesenteric margin involved by malignant neoplasm (finding)*

Distance of invasive carcinoma from closest margin: ___ mm OR ___ cm *[R-00481, 384891002] Distance of malignant neoplasm from closest margin (observable entity)*
Specify margin: ____ *[R-004EF, 396809007] surgical margin closest to malignant neoplasm (observable entity)*

LYMPHATIC (SMALL VESSEL) INVASION (L) (check all that apply) *[R-00404, 395715009]*
Status of lymphatic (small vessel) invasion by tumor (observable entity)
___ Absent *[G-F220, 44649003] L0 stage (finding)*
___ Present *[G-F221, 74139005] L1 stage (finding)*
    *___ Intramural *[F-02B82, 395718006] Lymphatic (small vessel) intramural invasion by*
tumor present (finding)
      *___ Extramural *[F-02B83, 395719003] Lymphatic (small vessel) extramural invasion*
by tumor present (finding)
___ Indeterminate *[G-F225, 33419001] LX stage (finding)*

VENOUS (LARGE VESSEL) INVASION (V) (check all that apply) *[R-00270, 371493002]*
Status of venous (large vessel) invasion by tumor (observable entity)
___ Absent *[G-F230, 40223008] V0 stage (finding)*
___ Present *[G-F539, 369732007] Venous (large vessel) invasion by tumor present (finding)*
    *___ Intramural *[G-F53A, 369733002] Venous (large vessel) intramural invasion by*
tumor present (finding)
    *___ Extramural *[G-F53B, 369734008] Venous (large vessel) extramural invasion by*
tumor present (finding)
___ Indeterminate *[G-F235, 6510002] VX stage (finding)*

*PERINEURAL INVASION *[R-0026D, 371513001] Status of perineural invasion by tumor*
(observable entity)
* ___ Absent *[G-F7A3, 370051000] Perineural invasion by tumor absent (finding)*
* ___ Present *[G-F538, 369731000] Perineural invasion by tumor present (finding)*

*TUMOR BORDER CONFIGURATION *[R-00260, 371502004] Tumor border configuration*
(observable entity)
* ___ Pushing *[G-F562, 369742009] Pushing tumor border (finding)*
* ___ Infiltrating *[G-F561, 369741002] Infiltrating tumor border, microscopic (finding)*

*INTRATUMORAL/PERITUMORAL LYMPHOCYTIC RESPONSE *[R-00407, 384604004]*
Status of intratumoral/peritumoral lymphocyte response (observable entity)
* ___ None *[F-D0193, 384601007] Intratumoral/peritumoral lymphocytic response absent*
(finding)
* ___ Mild to moderate *[F-D0194, 384602000] Intratumoral/peritumoral lymphocytic response*
mild to moderate (finding)
* ___ Marked (including Crohn-like response) *[R-00406, 384603005] Intratumoral/peritumoral*
lymphocytic response marked (finding)

*ADDITIONAL PATHOLOGIC FINDINGS (check all that apply) *[R-0025E, 371498006]*
Additional pathologic finding in tumor specimen (observable entity)
* ___ None identified *[F-02BB1, 395555008] No additional pathologic finding in tumor*
specimen (finding)
* ___ Adenoma(s) *[R-100D5, 399432003] Adenoma of large intestine (disorder)*
* ___ Chronic ulcerative proctocolitis *[D5-45281, 295046003] Ulcerative proctocolitis*
(disorder)

Appendix A: CAP Colon and Rectum Cancer Protocols and Checklists

*___ Crohn disease *[D5-41000, 34000006] Crohn's disease (disorder)*
*___ Dysplasia *[R-100D6, 399391008] Dysplasia of large intestine (disorder)*
*___ Other polyps (type[s]):__ *[R-100D7, 399505005] Polyp of large intestine (disorder)*
*___ Other (specify): ___ *not coded*

*COMMENT(S)

Copyright Notice:

This publication (product) incorporates SNOMED Clinical Terms® (SNOMED CT®) - The Systematized Nomenclature of Medicine Clinical Terms used by permission of the College of American Pathologists. © 2002- 2005 College of American Pathologists. SNOMED and SNOMED CT are registered trademarks of the College of American Pathologists, all rights reserved.

© 2002-2005 College of American Pathologists. SNOMED and SNOMED CT are registered trademarks of the College of American Pathologists, all rights reserved.

Appendix A: CAP Colon and Rectum Cancer Protocols and Checklists

Appendix B: Colon and Rectum Resection Checklist
Replacement of "Mesorectum" Section 4/04

*INTACTNESS OF MESORECTUM *[R-101CC, 408655002] Status of intactness of mesorectal specimen (observable entity)*
*___ Not applicable *[R-101CD, 408656001] Intactness of mesorectal specimen not applicable (finding)*
*___ Complete *[R-101CE, 408657005] Mesorectal specimen completely intact (finding)*
*___ Near complete *[R-101CF, 408658000] Mesorectal specimen nearly completely intact (finding)*
*___ Incomplete *[R-101D0, 408659008] Intactness of mesorectal specimen incomplete (finding)*

Appendix C: RPP-HL7 Segments Table

RPP HL7 Message Fields

HL7 ID Nbr	HL7 Name	HL7 Req	RPP Req	Cerner Uses	Calif. Uses	contents, format, or example	Data Type	RPP Max Len	Barry Gordon 11/29/04 Notes	NAACCR Data Item Name	NAACCR Data Item Nbr
MSH:01	Field Separator	R	R	R	R	|	ST				
MSH:02	Encoding Characters	R	R	R	R	"^~\&"	ST				
MSH:03	Sending Application	R	R	R	R		HD		Site-defined. We could use this to identify the sending software.		
MSH:04	Sending Facility	R	R	?	R	Path Facility ID # (CLIA #) Name^Code^CLIA e.g., UCIrvinePathology^05D0683594^CLIA	HD		Require that either number or name be filled in.		7010 & 7020
MSH:05	Receiving Application	O	O	Y	Y	e.g., "Cancer Registry Application"	HD				
MSH:06	Receiving Facility	O	O	Y	Y	"UCI" or "State Cancer Registry"	HD				
MSH:07	Date/Time of Message	O	R	R	R	YYYYMMDDHHMMSS	TS		HL7 requires, so we do	Date Case Report Exported	2110
MSH:09	Message Type	R	R	R	R	"ORU^R01"	CM				
MSH:10	Message Control ID	R	R	R	R	Locally defined internal counter. CDC suggests YYYYMMDDHHMMSS. Cerner: 13-digit	ST				
MSH:11	Processing ID	R	R	R	R	"P"	PT		For production		
MSH:12	Version ID	R	R	R	R	"2.3.1"	VID		CDC also uses 2.3.1		
MSH:13	Sequence Number	O	O								
MSH:16	App Ack Type	O	O						Are any acknowledgments expected?		
PID 01	Set ID - Patient ID	O	O	Y	Y	"1"	SI		Recommend that only one patient ID be used		

Appendix C: RPP-HL7 Segments Table

Report on the Reporting Pathology Protocols for Colon and Rectum Cancers Project   Version: 12/16/2005

HL7 ID Nbr	HL7 Name	HL7 Req	RPP Req	Cerner uses	Calif. Uses	contents, format, or example	Data Type	RPP Max Len	Notes	NAACCR Data Item Name	NAACCR Data Item Nbr
PID 03	Patient Identifier List	R	R	R	R	0310001^^^^MR^UCI&99999&CLIA~555441234^^^^SS. Cerner: "0nmmmmm^^^U"	CX		May contain both lab's and hospital's different id numbers, labeled PI and MR. Pt's SSN would be in another repeat, if available. Cerner uses MedRec # with 4th subfield containing code for hospital generating the number. Not all reports have MedRec #, but some kind of number is required here.	Medical Record Number	2300
PID 05	Patient Name	R	R	R	R	Lastname^Firstname^Middlename^Suffix^Prefix	XPN		Use only one complete name here. Cerner has period after MI.		2230, 40, 50
PID 07	Date of Birth	O	O	Y	O	YYYYMMDD	TS	8		Birth Date	240
PID 08	Sex	O	O	O	O	e.g. 'M'	IS	1		Sex	220
PID 09	Patient Alias	O	O	O	O	Lastname^Firstname^Middlename^Suffix^Prefix	XPN				2280
PID 10	Race	O	O	O	O	Race Code e.g., "B"	CE		Different codes than registry uses.		160
PID 11	Patient Address			O	O	street^other^city^state^zip^country	XAD				70,80,100,2330
PID 13	Phone Number-Home	O	O	O	O	Home Phone	XTN		Can include email address	Telephone Number	2360
PID 18	Patient Account No.		O	O	?	Currently missing in Cerner example			For billing. Maybe same as Visit #		
PID 19	SSN	O	O	O	O	Patient SSN Cerner uses dashes	ST	9	For backward compatibility. Also send in a repeat in PID -3	Social Security Number	2320

Appendix C: RPP-HL7 Segments Table

HL7 ID Nbr	HL7 Name	HL7 Req	RPP Req	Cerner uses	Calif. Uses	contents, format, or example	Data Type	RPP Max Len	Notes	NAACCR Data Item Name	NAACCR Data Item Nbr
PV1:01	Set ID - Patient Visit	R	R	R	R	"1"	SI				
PV1:02	Patient Class	R	O	O	Y	"I" or "O" for inpatient or outpatient	IS				
PV1:03	Assigned Patient Location	O	O	Y		Local codes; e.g., "000021^3W"	PL		For nursing, etc		
PV1:07	Attending Doctor	O	O	O	O		XCN		Cerner usually has local code and MD name for at least one of these 4		
PV1:08	Referring Doctor		O	O			XCN				
PV1:09	Consulting Doctor		O	O			XCN				
PV1:17	Admitting Doctor		O	O			XCN				
PV1:18	Patient Type		O	O		Cerner: local codes; e.g., "D"	IS		e.g., inpatient, outpatient		
PV1:19	Visit Number	O	O	O		Cerner uses alphanumeric codes from ADT; e.g., "nnnnn"	CX		Encounter number, site specific		
PV1:44	Admit Date/Time		O	O	O	YYYYMMDDHHMM	TS				
PV1:45	Discharge Date/Time		O	O	O	YYYYMMDDHHMM	TS				
ORC:01	Order Control	R	R	R	R	CN or RE	ST		CDC uses "CN" for "combined result" Cerner uses RE for "observations to follow"		
ORC:02	Placer Order Number	C	O	O		alphanumeric	EI		Depends on hospital infor system. Used in OBR-02 as well		
ORC:03	Filler Order #	C	R	Y	Y	The accession number pathologists refer to; e.g., "SS96-nnnnn^CoPathPlus"	EI		The CoPath accession number. Use OBR segment. Pathologists use this to refer to.		

Page 78 of 124

Appendix C: RPP-HL7 Segments Table

Report on the Reporting Pathology Protocols for Colon and Rectum Cancers Project   Version: 12/16/2005

HL7 ID Nbr	HL7 Name	HL7 Req	RPP Req	Cerner uses	Calif. Uses	contents, format, or example	Data Type	RPP Max Len	Notes	NAACCR Data Item Name	NAACCR Data Item Nbr
ORC:04	Order Status			Y		"CM"	ST		Skip		
ORC:09	Date/Time Transaction		O	Y		Accession Date/Time	TS		Cerner: date/time accessioned		
ORC:10	Entered by		O	Y		Manager^system	XCN		Accessioner		
ORC:12	Ordering Provider		O	Y		Cerner Uses e.g., nnnnn^Welby Jr ^Marcus	XCN		Submitting MD. Use OBR-16 segment too		
ORC:21	Ordering Facility Name	R	R	R	R	Name^^Number; e.g., "UHC"	XON		May use AHA or ACoS number. Cerner uses client codes		
ORC:22	Ordering Facility Address	O	O	O		street^other^city^state^zip^country	XAD		If available		
ORC:23	Ordering Facility Phone Number	O	O	O		555-5555	XTN		If available	Can include email	
ORC:24	Ordering Provider Address	O	O	O	O		XAD		If available		
OBR 01	Set ID - Order	O	O	O	O	"1"	SI				
OBR 02	Placer Order Number	C	O	O			EI		Also in ORC-02. California wants to use the second segment of this field to track the location of the facility requesting the path report.		
OBR 03	Filler Order #	R	R	Y	Y	Cerner: XXYY-999999	EI	20	Contains specimen accession number	Path–slide report number	7090
OBR 04	Universal Service ID	R	R	Y	Y	Locally defined. Could be SNOMED code for "surgical procedure." Cerner: "UHC Surgical Pathology Department" California: SP	CE		Broadly identifies source of specimen. OBX3 has specifics. OBR-44 will contain the protocol checklist ID		

Appendix C: RPP-HL7 Segments Table

HL7 ID Nbr	HL7 Name	HL7 Req	RPP Req	Cerner uses	Calif. Uses	contents, format, or example	Data Type	RPP Max Len	Notes	NAACCR Data Item Name	NAACCR Data Item Nbr
OBR 07	Observation Date/Time	R	R	R	R	YYYYMMDDHHMM	TS	8	Date/time path specimen was collected or obtained. If actual surgery date is unknown, use date accessioned so this is never empty	Path–date of specimen collection	7320
OBR 10	Collector Identifier	O	O	O	N		XCN		Q from Epath group - Add this to capture the surgeon ID? Answer: RPP doesn't need, because it is the same as OBR16 Ordering Provide, who is the surgeon.		
OBR 14	Specimen Received Date/Time	C	O	O	N	YYYYMMDDHHMM	TS		Actual login time at the diagnostic lab. Accession date.		
OBR 15	Specimen Source	O	O	Y	Y	User Defined. CA: TISS (HL7 Table 70) Cerner: uses locally defined tbl	CM		Details will appear in an OBX		
OBR 16	Ordering Provider	O	O	Y	Y	License #/Physician (Attending^Lastname^Firstname^ Middlename. Require UPIN code Is attending MD different than ordering MD?	XCN		Both license # and physician name. Also in ORC-12. Cannot require because may be a clinic, not a specific MD. This is the surgeon, not necessarily the attending MD, which is in PV1-7. The NAACCR write-up is wrong	Ordering client/physician-license number	7100, 7120, 7130 & 7190

Appendix C: RPP-HL7 Segments Table

Report on the Reporting Pathology Protocols for Colon and Rectum Cancers Project   Version: 12/16/2005

HL7 ID Nbr	HL7 Name	HL7 Req	RPP Req	Cerner uses	Calif. Uses	contents, format, or example	Data Type	RPP Max Len	Notes	NAACCR Data Item Name	NAACCR Data Item Nbr
OBR 17	Order Call Back Telephone #	O	O	O		(510) 555-1212 rarely available	XTN	10	Can include email address	Ordering client/physician -telephone	7180
OBR 22	Results Rpt/Status Change - D/T	C	O	Y	Y		TS		Date/time results signed out		
OBR 24	Diagnosis Serv Sect ID	O	O	Y	Y	"SP" surgical pathology. Cerner uses same	ID		Not listed in CDC guide		
OBR 25	Results Status	C	O	O	O	"F" for final report. "C" if amendment or correction	ID		Code from HL7 table 0123. We might want to be able to accept corrections also		
OBR 29	Parent	O	O	O	O				Points back to earlier report on same sample.		
OBR 31	Reason for Study	O	O			Not available	CE		CDC uses		
OBR 32	Principal Result Interpretor	O	R	Y	Y	Primary pathologist License#^Lastname^Firstname^Middlename^suffix. Cerner uses	XCN		License number may be UPIN or locally defined. (not mentioned in CDC guide)	Path--reporting pathologist name, license	7260-7310
OBR 44	Procedure Code	O	R	Y	Y	SNOMED's code for the checklist used (e.g., R-10118)			Instead, we will use it to define which checklist is used. Do we put CAP version here too?		

Appendix C: RPP-HL7 Segments Table

HL7 ID Nbr	HL7 Name	HL7 Req	RPP Req	Cerner Uses	Calif. Uses	contents, format, or example	Data Type	RPP Max Len	Notes	NAACCR Data Item Name	NAACCR Data Item Nbr
OBR 45	Procedure Code Modifier		?						Do we put CAP version here? Propose format for this; e.g., Jan04 Waiting for SNOMED to confirm that they will change the checklist concept ID for each semiannual release. If so, we can use OBR44 to track protocol changes in concepts.		
OBX:01	Set ID	O	R	R	R	The order of OBXs is not defined	SI		Allows receiver to maintain relational aspects of message		
OBX:02	Value Type	C	R	R	R	"CE" or "ST" or "TX" or "FT" or CWE or NM	ID				
OBX:03	Observation ID	R	R	R	R	LOINC or local ID that corresponds with the OBX-5 values or text	CE				
OBX:04	Observation Sub-ID	C		X	X	If the OBX contains source/part information (text type = ANT)	ST				
OBX:05	Observation Value	C	R	R	R	Coded entries and text	CE, TX		The text items that we use are clinical history and final DX blocks. final DX will be used to document results from pieces that are not colon/rectum		
OBX:06	Units	O	O	O	O	e.g., mm	CE		For numeric items		

Appendix C: RPP-HL7 Segments Table

Appendix D: RPP-OBX Segments Table

OBX results: Questions with proposed SNOMED and LOINC codes for colorectal checklist

RPP Item #	Proposed Item Name for Messaging	CAP Checklist Item Name	LOINC Code	Data Type	Screen Order			Re-quired?	Allow Multiple Answers?	SNOMED Code	SNOMED Concept Description	BG Notes
					Colon and Rectum Poly-pectomy	Rectum: Local Excision	Colon and Rectum Resection					
	CAP Checklist or Document Name											We will use OBR to identify checklist, so don't need an OBX element
1	Specimen type	Specimen type	33722-0	CWE	Automatically send the "polyp" value	1	1	Yes	No	371439000	Specimen type (observable entity)	Make a CWE field to handle text of "other"
2	Specimen length	Length	33723-8	NM			2	No	No	384606002	Length of specimen (observable entity)	This is used to code the length of any of the specimen types
3	Specimen Type—Other (text)	Specimen type—other (text)	33724-6	ST			3	No				Use CWE type in field 01 for this text
4	Tumor site	Tumor site	33725-3	CE	1	4	4	Yes		263601005	Tumor site (observable entity)	
5	Tumor configuration	Tumor configuration	33726-1	CWE		7	5	No		371500007	Tumor configuration (observable entity)	
6	Tumor Configuration—Other (text)	Other (specify) not coded	33727-9	ST			6	No				Use above CWE
7	Tumor size (greatest dimension)	Tumor size greatest dimension	33728-7	NM		8	7	Yes		371479009	Tumor size, largest N21 dimension (observable entity)	

Barry Gordon 8/19/2004

Appendix D: RPP-OBX Segments Table

Report on the Reporting Pathology Protocols for Colon and Rectum Cancers Project

RPP Item #	Proposed Item Name for Messaging	CAP Checklist Item Name	LOINC Code	Data Type	Colon and Rectum Poly-pectomy	Rectum: Local Excision	Colon and Rectum Resection	Re-quired?	Allow Multiple Answers?	SNOMED Code	SNOMED Concept Description	BG Notes
8	Tumor size additional dimensions [2nd]	Additional dimensions	33729-5	NM		9	8	No	Yes	395512009	Tumor size, additional dimension (observable entity)	LOINC wants us to use repeats rather than sub-IDs to handle 2nd and 3rd dimension
9	Tumor size additional dimensions [3d]	Additional dimensions	33729-5	NM		10	9	No	Yes	395512009	Tumor size, additional dimension (observable entity)	LOINC wants us to use repeats rather than sub-IDs to handle 2nd and 3rd dimension
10	Intactness of mesorectum	Intactness of mesorectum	33730-3	CE			10	No		408865002	Status of intactness of mesorectal specimen (observable entity)	What do you send if no invasion of mesorectum? Answer: don't send this item
11	Histologic type	Histologic type	31205-8	CWE	7	11	11	Yes		371441004	Histologic type (observable entity)	
~~12~~	~~Histologic Type Text (Other)~~	Other (specify)	33731-1	ST	8	12	12	No				
13	Histologic Grade (hi/low)	Histologic Grade	33732-9	CWE	9	13	13	yes		371469007	Histologic grade (observable entity)	
~~52~~	~~Histologic Grade Text~~	Other (specify)	CWE in RPP13					No				Added 7/1/03 checklist
14	Extent of invasion primary tumor (pT)	Primary tumor (pT)	21899-0	CE		14	14	Yes		384625004	pT Category (observable entity)	
15	Regional lymph nodes (pN)	Regional lymph nodes (pN)	21900-6	CE		15	15	Some		371494008	pN Category (observable entity)	pN category
16	Number of nodes examined	Number examined	21894-1	NM		16	16	Some		372309006	Number of regional lymph nodes examined (observable entity)	

Appendix D: RPP-OBX Segments Table

RPP Item #	Proposed Item Name for Messaging	CAP Checklist Item Name	LOINC Code	Data Type	Colon and Rectum Poly-pectomy	Rectum: Local Excision	Colon and Rectum Resection	Re-quired?	Allow Multiple Answers?	SNOMED Code	SNOMED Concept Description	BG Notes
17	Number of nodes involved	Number involved	21893-3	NM		17	17	Some		372308003	Number of regional lymph nodes involved (observable entity)	
18	Distant metastasis (pM)	Distant metastasis (pM)	21901-4	CE			18	Some		371497001	Stage of distant metastasis of tumor (observable entity)	
19	Site(s) of distant metastasis (text)	Specify sites(s)	33733-7	ST			19	No		385421009	Site of distant metastasis (observable entity)	
20	Proximal margin	Status of surgical proximal margin	33734-5	CE			20	Some		372439002	Status of surgical proximal margin involvement by tumor (observable entity)	
21	Distal margin	Status of surgical distal margin	33735-2	CE			21	Some		372440000	Status of surgical distal margin involvement by tumor (observable entity)	
22	Circumferential (radial) margin	Circumferential (radial) margin	33736-0	CE			22	Some		384618006	Status of surgical circumferential margin involvement by tumor (observable entity)	
23	Distance of invasive carcinoma from closest margin	Distance of invasive carcinoma from closest margin	33737-8	NM			23	Some		384891002	Distance of malignant neoplasm from closest margin (observable entity)	Convert to mm in message. LOINC term is "distance of tumor"

Appendix D: RPP-OBX Segments Table

Report on the Reporting Pathology Protocols for Colon and Rectum Cancers Project   Version: 12/16/2005

RPP Item #	Proposed Item Name for Messaging	CAP Checklist Item Name	LOINC Code	Data Type	Colon and Rectum Poly-pectomy	Rectum: Local Excision	Colon and Rectum Resection	Re-quired?	Allow Multiple Answers?	SNOMED Code	SNOMED Concept Description	BG Notes
24	Specify closest margin	Specify margin	33738-6	CE			24	Some		396809007	Specimen margin closest to malignant neoplasm (observable entity)	We need to agree on the values for this coded field
25	Lymphatic (small vessel) Invasion	Lymphatic (small) vessel invasion (L)	33739-4	CE	16	24	25	Some	Yes	395715009	Status of lymphatic (small vessel) invasion by tumor (observable entity)	
26	Venous (large vessel) invasion	Venous (large) vessel invasion (V)	33740-2	CE	17	25	26	Some	Yes	371493002	Status of tumor invasion of venous (large) vessel (observable entity)	
27	Perineural invasion	Perineural invasion	33741-0	CE		26	27	No		371513001	Status of tumor perineural invasion (observable entity)	
28	Tumor border configuration	Tumor border configuration	33742-8	CE		27	28	No		371502004	Tumor border configuration (observable entity)	
29	Intratumoral/ peritumoral lymphocytic response	Intratumoral/peritumoral lymphocytic response	33743-6	CE		28	29	No		384604004	Status of intratumoral/peri tumoral lymphocyte response (observable entity)	
30	Additional pathologic findings	Additional pathologic findings	33744-4	CWE	19	29	30	No	Yes	371498006	Additional pathologic finding in tumor specimen (observable entity)	

Appendix D: RPP-OBX Segments Table

Report on the Reporting Pathology Protocols for Colon and Rectum Cancers Project   Version: 12/16/2005

RPP Item #	Proposed Item Name for Messaging	CAP Checklist Item Name	LOINC code	Data type	Colon and Rectum Poly-pectomy	Rectum: Local Excision	Colon and Rectum Resection	Re-quired?	Allow Multiple Answers?	SNOMED Code	SNOMED Concept Description	BG Notes
31	Other polyps—text	Other polyps—text	33745-1	ST		30	31	No				
32	Other pathologic findings (text)	Other (specify)	33746-9	ST	20	31	32	No				We made up name
33	Additional text on CAP checklist	Comment(s) not coded	22638-1	ST	21	32	33	No		409770001	Narrative comments on pathology specimen (observable entity)	I renamed it from "comment (s) not coded"
34	Number of pieces	Number of pieces	33747-7	NM		3		No		395558005	Number of pieces in fragmented specimen (observable entity)	
35	Distance from anal verge	Distance from anal verge	33748-5	NM		5		No		371490004	Distance of tumor from anal verge (observable entity)	cm
36	Distance from anal verge unknown	Distance from anal verge unknown	33749-3	CE		6		No		372298005	Distance of tumor from anal verge unknown (finding)	Code unknown separately from above item—or is there a way to do this in the numeric HL7 field? Check v 2.4 & 2.5 BG
37	~~Margins cannot be assessed~~	~~Margin~~	~~33750-1~~	~~CE~~	~~11~~	~~18?~~		~~No~~		~~82868003~~		No longer needed—there is a separate response for each margin

Appendix D: RPP-OBX Segments Table

RPP Item #	Proposed Item Name for Messaging	CAP Checklist Item Name	LOINC Code	Data Type	Colon and Rectum Poly-pectomy	Rectum: Local Excision	Colon and Rectum Resection	Re-quired?	Allow Multiple Answers?	SNOMED Code	Snomed Concept Description	BG Notes
38	Mucosal/lateral margin	Mucosal/lateral margin	33751-9	CE	15	19		Some		384786009	Status of surgical lateral (mucosal/mural) margin involvement by tumor (observable entity)	This now joined with item that was R-00475 (#49)
39	Distance of carcinoma from closest lateral margin	Distance of carcinoma from closest lateral margin	33752-7	NM		20		Depends		385393002	Distance of malignant neoplasm from closest lateral margin (observable entity)	mm. This different than RPP 23 because it is specific to lateral margin
40	Lateral margin location text	Specify location, if possible not coded	33753-5	ST		21		No				Same field used for uninvolved and involved, but it's OK because they are mutually exclusive
41	Deep margin status	Deep margin	33754-3	CE	13	22		Some		395543002	Status of deep (radial) surgical tumor margin involvement (observable entity)	
42	Distance of invasive carcinoma from deep margin	Distance of invasive carcinoma from margin	33755-0	NM	14	23		Some		385390003	Distance of malignant neoplasm from deep margin (observable entity)	mm
43	Polyp size greatest dimension	Greatest dimension	33756-8	NM	2			Yes		372259000	Polyp size, largest dimension (observable entity)	

Appendix D: RPP-OBX Segments Table

Report on the Reporting Pathology Protocols for Colon and Rectum Cancers Project   Version: 12/16/2005

RPP Item #	Proposed Item Name for Messaging	CAP Checklist Item Name	LOINC Code	Data Type	Colon and Rectum Poly-pectomy	Rectum: Local Excision	Colon and Rectum Resection	Re-quired?	Allow Multiple Answers?	SNOMED Code	Snomed Concept Description	BG Notes
44	Polyp size additional dimensions [2nd]	Polyp size additional dimensions	33757-6	NM	3			No		395509006	Polyp size, additional dimension (observable entity)	Not mentioned in 11/18/02 list
45	Polyp size additional dimensions [3rd]	Polyp size additional dimensions	33757-6	NM	4			No		395509006	Polyp size, additional dimension (observable entity)	
46	Polyp configuration	Polyp configuration		CE	5			Yes		371501006	Polyp configuration (observable entity)	LOINC suggested we use the "tumor configuration" item RPP05 and reference polyp answers only in polypectomies. SNOMED says they are different concepts. We will us SNOMED for now
47	Polyp stalk length	Stalk length	33758-4	NM	6			No?		395511002	Stalk length (observable entity)	
48	Extent of invasion	Extent of invasion	33759-2	CE	10			Yes		371487005	Tumor extent of invasion (observable entity)	Not p codes
49	Mucosal margin	Mucosal margin	33760-0								status of surgical mucosal margin involvement by tumor	Removed, merged with #38
50	Venous/Lymphatic (Small) Vessel Invasion (V/L)	Venous/Lymphatic (Small) Vessel Invasion (V/L)	33761-8	CE	16	-	-	Yes		371492007	Status of lymphatic (small vessel) invasion by tumor (observable entity)	No longer needed–same concept across all 3 protocols

Appendix D: RPP-OBX Segments Table

RPP Item #	Proposed Item Name for Messaging	CAP Checklist Item Name	LOINC Code	Data Type	Colon and Rectum Poly-pectomy	Rectum: Local Excision	Colon and Rectum Resection	Re-quired?	Allow Multiple Answers?	SNOMED code	Snomed Concept Description	BG Notes
51	Specimen integrity	Specimen integrity	R-100A8	CE		2				397191008		Keep concept separate from # of pieces. Calif. may add inter-field edit
53	Tumor size cannot be determined	Tumor size cannot be determined	F-02BBE	CE		10A	9A			396919000		Separate item in message. Can generate 999s in size at cancer registry.
54	Type of polyp	Type of polyp in which invasive carcinoma arose		CE	18					406126002	Type of polyp in which invasive carcinoma arose (observable entity)	Added Jan 2004
55	Mesenteric margin	Mesenteric margin		CE			22A	No		405981000	Status of surgical mesenteric margin involvement by tumor (observable entity)	Added Jan 2004

Appendix D: RPP-OBX Segments Table

Appendix E: RPP Alpha Test Messages - 2004
De-identified and Edited – 2005.01.20

MSH|^~\&|CoPathPlus||Cancer Registry Application|State Cancer
Registry|20040204180600||ORU^R01|1700000000170|P|2.3.1
PID|1||01111111^^^U||PATIENT^TEST1^C.||19550401|M||ZEO-1|||||||||111-11-1111
PV1|1||000021^3W|||||||||||||||D|858473|AASU|||||||||||||||||||||||||200401011200
ORC|RE||SS96-24610^CoPathPlus||CM||||200401251413|^Manager^System||01302^SMITH
Jr^JOHN||||||||||UHC|11100 Euclid Avenue^^Cleveland^OH^44106-5000^United States|555-
5555|Wearn 233 Stop 5066^UHC/DEPT MED-GASTRO^CLEVELAND^OH^44106^United
States
OBR|1||SS96-24610^CoPathPlus|^UHC Surgical Pathology
Department||||199612190000|||||||199612190000|SDSTY-
369|01302||||||200401271238||SP|F|||||||12198^WELBY^MARCUS|12198^WELBY^MARCUS||||||
||||||R-10117^^^SNOMED-CT
OBX|1|CE|33722-0^SpecimenType^LN||235340004^Polypectomy - large intestine^SNOMED-
CT||||||F
OBX|2|CE|33725-3^ColonTumorSite^LN||14742008^NotSpecified^SNOMED-CT||||||F
OBX|3|CE|00000-0^ColonInvPolyp^LN||61722000^Tubulovillous adenoma^SNOMED-CT||||||F
OBX|4|CE|33744-4^ColonAddFind^LN||395555008^AddlFindingsNone^SNOMED-CT||||||F
OBX|5|CE|33756-8^ColonPolypSize^LN||397361006^CannotBeDetermined^SNOMED-CT||||||F
OBX|6|CE|^ColonPolypConf||395528004^Fragmented^SNOMED-CT||||||F
OBX|7|CE|31205-8^ColonHistoType^LN||35917007^Adenocarcinoma^SNOMED-CT||||||F
OBX|8|CE|33732-9^ColonHistGrade^LN||395529007^LowHistologicGrade^SNOMED-CT||||||F
OBX|9|CE|33759-2^ColonInvasion^LN||395532005^CannotBeDetermined^SNOMED-CT||||||F
OBX|10|NM|33755-
0^DeepMarginDistanceFromInvCarc^LN||2^DeepMarginDistanceFromInvCarc|mm|||||F
OBX|11|CE|33739-4^ColonInvasionL^LN||44649003^LymphaticInvasionAbsent^SNOMED-
CT||||||F
OBX|12|CE|33740-2^ColonInvasionV^LN||40223008^VenousInvasionAbsent^SNOMED-
CT||||||F

MSH|^~\&|CoPathPlus||Cancer Registry Application|State Cancer
Registry|20040205084300||ORU^R01|1700000000169|P|2.3.1
PID|1||02222222^^^U||PATIENT^TEST2^J.||19140401|M||ZEO-1|||||||||222-22-2222
PV1|1||0NSU^14N-
6||||12564^DAVE^LASTNAME|28122^JOE^TEST|10000^MARY^TESTING||||||||13625^LNA
ME-SURNAME^NANCY|8|987654|MM2A|||||||||||||||||||||||||200401010000
ORC|RE||SS01-
26488^CoPathPlus||CM||||200401131614|^Manager^System||45599^JOE^SMITH||||||||UHC|1110
0 Euclid Avenue^^Cleveland^OH^44106-5000^United States|555-5555|870 W MAIN
ST^^GENEVA^OH^44041^United States
OBR|1||SS01-26488^CoPathPlus|^UHC Surgical Pathology
Department||||200110160000|||||||200110170000|SDSTY-
348|45599||||||200401271230||SP|F|||||||12198^WELBY^MARCUS|12198^WELBY^MARCUS||||||
||||||R-10119^^^SNOMED-CT
OBX|1|CE|33722-0^ColonSpecType^LN||122648004^RightHemicolectomy^SNOMED-CT||||||F

OBX|2|CE|21900-
6^ColonNodes^LN||395711000^pN1:MetastasisIn1to3LymphNodes^SNOMED-CT||||||F
OBX|3|NM|21894-1^NumberOfNodesExamined^LN||0^NumberOfNodesExamined||||||F
OBX|4|NM|21893-3^NumberOfNodesInvolved^LN||9^NumberOfNodesInvolved||||||F
OBX|5|CE|21901-4^ColonMetastasis^LN||17076002^pMX:CannotBeAssessed^SNOMED-
CT||||||F
OBX|6|CE|33734-
5^ProximalMarginUninvolved^LN||384614008^ProximalMarginUninvolved^SNOMED-CT||||||F
OBX|7|CE|33735-
2^DistalMarginUninvolved^LN||384623006^DistalMarginUninvolved^SNOMED-CT||||||F
OBX|8|CE|33736-
0^CircumfMarginNotApplicable^LN||384619003^CircumfMarginNotApplicable^SNOMED-
CT||||||F
OBX|9|CWE|00000-
0^MesentericMarginUninvolved^LN||405984008^MesentericMarginUninvolved^SNOMED-
CT||||||F
OBX|10|CE|33739-4^ColonInvasionL^LN||44649003^LymphaticInvasionAbsent^SNOMED-
CT||||||F
OBX|11|CE|33740-2^ColonInvasionV^LN||40223008^VenousInvasionAbsent^SNOMED-
CT||||||F
OBX|12|NM|33722-0^ColonSpecType^LN||19^LengthOfSpecimen|cm||||||F
OBX|13|CE|33741-0^ColonPerineural^LN||370051000^PerineuralInvasionAbsent^SNOMED-
CT||||||F
OBX|14|CE|33742-8^ColonTumerBordr^LN||369741002^TumorBorderInfiltrating^SNOMED-
CT||||||F
OBX|15|CE|33743-
6^ColonLymphoResp^LN||384601007^Intra/PeriLymphResponseNone^SNOMED-CT||||||F
OBX|16|CE|33744-4^ColonAddFind^LN||399432003^AdenomaLargeIntestine^SNOMED-
CT||||||F
OBX|17|ST|33746-9^OtherAddlFinding^LN||Mesentery dissected twice for lymph
nodes.^OtherAddlFinding||||||F
OBX|18|CE|33725-3^ColonTumorSite^LN||51342009^RightAscendingColon^SNOMED-
CT||||||F
OBX|19|CE|33726-1^ColonTumorConf^LN||369752008^Infiltrative^SNOMED-CT||||||F
OBX|20|NM|33728-7^GreatestDimension^LN||3.5^GreatestDimension|cm||||||F
OBX|21|CE|33730-
3^ColonMesorectum^LN||408656001^MesorectumNotApplicable^SNOMED-CT||||||F
OBX|22|CE|31205-8^ColonHistoType^LN||35917007^Adenocarcinoma^SNOMED-CT||||||F
OBX|23|CE|33732-9^ColonHistGrade^LN||395529007^LowHistologicGrade^SNOMED-
CT||||||F
OBX|24|CE|21899-0^ColonPriTumor^LN||395707006^pT3:TumorInvasion^SNOMED-CT||||||F

MSH|^~\&|CoPathPlus||Cancer Registry Application|State Cancer
Registry|20040205084300||ORU^R01|1700000000168|P|2.3.1
PID|1||03333333^^^U||PATIENT^TEST3^F.||19210401|M||ZEO-1|||||||||333-33-3333

PV1|1||0CCT^5W-
3|||||19455^THOMAS^SURNAME|26110^LASTNAME^DAVID|||||||||36825^TESTING^STEPH
EN|D|868686|AASU|||||||||||||||||||||||||200401010000
ORC|RE||SS96-
14705^CoPathPlus||CM||||200401251401|^Manager^System||03048^LNAME^ROBERT|||||||||UH
C|11100 Euclid Avenue^^Cleveland^OH^44106-5000^United States|555-5555|UHC/DEPT
SUR-GENERAL^^CLEVELAND^OH^44106^United States
OBR|1||SS96-14705^CoPathPlus|^UHC Surgical Pathology
Department||||199607290000||||||||199607290000|SDSTY-
183|03048||||||200401271142||SP|F|||||||12198^WELBY^MARCUS|12198^WELBY^MARCUS||||||
||||||R-10118^^SNOMED-CT
OBX|1|CE|33722-0^SpecimenType^LN||287784004^LocalExcisionOfRectum^SNOMED-
CT||||||F
OBX|2|CE|33725-3^TumorSite^LN||34402009^RectumStructure^SNOMED-CT||||||F
OBX|3|CE|00000-0^ColonSpecIntegr^LN||397315006^SpecimenIntact^SNOMED-CT||||||F
OBX|4|NM|33755-
0^DeepMarginDistanceFromInvCarc^LN||2^DeepMarginDistanceFromInvCarc|mm|||||F
OBX|5|CE|33739-4^ColonInvasionL^LN||44649003^LymphaticInvasionAbsent^SNOMED-
CT||||||F
OBX|6|CE|33740-2^ColonInvasionV^LN||40223008^VenousInvasionAbsent^SNOMED-CT||||||F
OBX|7|CE|33741-0^ColonPerineural^LN||370051000^PerineuralInvasionAbsent^SNOMED-
CT||||||F
OBX|8|CE|33742-8^ColonTumerBordr^LN||369741002^TumorBorderInfiltrating^SNOMED-
CT||||||F
OBX|9|CE|33743-
6^ColonLymphoResp^LN||384601007^Intra/PeriLymphResponseNone^SNOMED-CT||||||F
OBX|10|CE|33744-4^ColonAddFind^LN||395555008^AddlFindingsNone^SNOMED-CT||||||F
OBX|11|CE|33749-
3^DistanceFromAnalVergeUnknown^LN||372298005^DistanceFromAnalVergeUnknown^SNO
MED-CT||||||F
OBX|12|CE|33726-1^ColonTumorConf^LN||369752008^Infiltrative^SNOMED-CT||||||F
OBX|13|NM|33728-7^GreatestDimension^LN||1^GreatestDimension|cm|||||F
OBX|14|CE|31205-8^ColonHistoType^LN||35917007^Adenocarcinoma^SNOMED-CT||||||F
OBX|15|CE|33732-9^ColonHistGrade^LN||395529007^LowHistologicGrade^SNOMED-
CT||||||F
OBX|16|CE|21899-
0^ColonPriTumor^LN||373200003^pT1:TumorInvadesSubmucosa^SNOMED-CT||||||F
OBX|17|CE|21900-6^ColonNodes^LN||54452005^pNX:CannotBeAssessed^SNOMED-CT||||||F
OBX|18|CE|33751-
9^LateralMarginInvolvedCISAdenom^LN||397189000^LateralMarginInvolvedCISAdenom^SN
OMED-CT||||||F

MSH|^~\&|CNET_RPP|22D9999999|CNET_CAS|UCI_CancerRegistry|200312011159||ORU\S\
R01|20031201120000|P|2.3.1
PID||1|3000021^^^^PI^UCIPathology&99D1234567&CLIA~MR777777^^^^PT^UCI_Hospital
&01334455&CA||Testcase^Numberten^^^^^^L-

Appendix E: RPP Alpha Test Messages – 2004

Legal||19250131000000000|M|||||||||||999999999PV1|1|I|||||^Welby^MarcusORC|CN||3000021^Co Path|||||||||||||||||UCIrvine

OBR|1||S3000021|X|||20030101000000000|||||||||1234567^Welby^M^^^Dr^MD|||||||||||||||1234&Lin &Fritz&&&&MD|||||||||||235340004^Polypectomy CAP Protocol^SNOMED-CT

OBX|1|ST|33722-0^Specimen Type^LN||122645001\S\specimen from large intestine obtained by excisioinal biopsy (polypectomy) of lesion\S\SNOMED-CT|||||F

OBX|2|CE|33725-3^Tumor Site^LN||72592005^Splenic flexure^SNOMED-CT|||||F

OBX|3|NM|33756-8^Polyp Size Greatest Dimension^LN||3|^CM|||||F

OBX|4|NM|33757-6^Polyp Size Additional Dimensions^LN||2|^CM|||||F

OBX|5||371501006^Polyp configuration^SNOMED-CT||395498009\S\Pedunculated with stalk\S\SNOMED-CT|||||F

OBX|6|CE|31205-8^Histologic Type^LN||35917007^Adenocarcinoma^SNOMED-CT|||||F

OBX|7|CWE|33732-9^Histologic Grade (hi/low)^LN||395530002^High-grade^SNOMED-CT|||||F

OBX|8|CE|33759-2^Extent of invasion^LN||395532005^Cannot be determined^SNOMED-CT|||||F

OBX|9|CE|37754-3^Deep margin^LN||399652005^Cannot be assessed^SNOMED-CT|||||F

OBX|10|CE|33751-9^Mucosal/lateral margin^LN||405980004^Cannot be assessed^SNOMED-CT|||||F

OBX|11|CE|33739-4^Lymphatic invasion^LN||33419001^Indeterminate^SNOMED-CT|||||F

OBX|12|CE|33740-2^Venous invasion^LN||6510002^ Indeterminate^SNOMED-CT|||||F

OBX|33|ST|22638-1^Additional Text on CAP checklist^LN||entered by kda|||||F

Appendix F: Message: Questions and Answers
Compiled June 2004 – Updated July 2004

Note: These questions were compiled from the RPP meeting highlights (minutes) from October 2003 through January 2004. The questions are grouped under three basic headings: HL7 Message, Unresolved, and Checklist. The questions are numbered sequentially under each category and the associated RPP meeting or other source is noted with [ ] brackets.

HL7 Message

1 - Question: Should there be one OBR segment for each CAP cancer protocols checklist. Specifically, should there be a separate OBR for the clinical history or the narrative final diagnosis?
Discussion: There was a reference to the CDC-NPCR document, Implementation Guide for Transmission of Laboratory-Based Reporting of Public Health Information using Version 2.3.1 of the Health Level Seven (HL7) Standard Protocol, Implementation Guide Update April 21, 2003. The focus of this guide is in the area of infectious disease and notes that the scope of an OBR segment is generic for a laboratory report with different OBX segments. Presently, the Co-Path standards use multiple OBR segments for special stains.
Decision: Each message should contain a single OBR segment to correspond to the specific laboratory and appropriate CAP checklist name with the associated SNOMED codes.
[Reporting Pathology Protocols (RPP) Messaging Work Group on October 1, 2003]

2 - Question: Should we allow more than one OBR?
Discussion: For this study, we had already agreed to use only one OBR; however this issue may need more thought. Conceivably, a report could contain two different sources of tissue.
Decision: We will only use one OBR. When and if the need for more than one ORB becomes apparent from a real situation we will reassess.
[Reporting Pathology Protocols (RPP) Messaging Work Group on January 7, 2004]

3 - Question: Does the order of the OBX segments in the message matter?
Discussion: The order in the California system is based on the RPP Item Number in the Excel file spreadsheet, while the order with Cerner is based on the CAP checklist. Each OBX segment will contain unique identifiers.
Decision: The order should not matter. There is no need for consistency in this area.
[Reporting Pathology Protocols (RPP) Messaging Work Group on October 29, 2003]

4 - Question: The OBX counters on the California sample message vary from those on the Cerner sample message. Should the OBX counters refer to the same segment?
Discussion: Having the same OBX counters would make comparisons between the two sample messages easier. Many of the examples in HL7 documentation use the OBX counter similar to those used in the Cerner sample message.
Decision: The OBX counters should be sequential.
[Reporting Pathology Protocols (RPP) Messaging Work Group on December 4, 2003]

5 - Question: Which OBR attributes are needed?
Discussion: See Meeting Comment column.

Appendix F: Message: Questions and Answers

OBR attributes

SEQ	LEN	DT	OTP	ITEM #	ELEMENT NAME	Meeting Comment:
1	4	SI	O	00237	Set ID - OBR	Fill as a 1
2	22	EI	C	00216	Placer Order Number	
3	22	EI	C	00217	Filler Order Number +	This attribute is needed, tied to the accession number
4	200	CE	R	00238	Universal Service ID	Possible use, unclear at present
5	2	ID	X	00239	Priority	
6	26	TS	X	00240	Requested Date/time	Needed
7	26	TS	C	00241	Observation Date/Time #	
8	26	TS	O	00242	Observation End Date/Time #	
9	20	CQ	O	00243	Collection Volume *	
10	60	XCN	O	00244	Collector Identifier *	
11	1	ID	O	00245	Specimen Action Code *	
12	60	CE	O	00246	Danger Code	
13	300	ST	O	00247	Relevant Clinical Info.	
14	26	TS	C	00248	Specimen Received Date/Time *	Needed
15	300	CM	O	00249	Specimen Source *	Needed
16	80	XCN	O	00226	Ordering Provider	Cancer registrars need this information. Cerner uses the Universal Physician Identification Number (UPIN)
17	40	XTN	O	00250	Order Callback Phone Number	Needed
18	60	ST	O	00251	Placer Field 1	
19	60	ST	O	00252	Placer Field 2	
20	60	ST	O	00253	Filler Field 1 +	
21	60	ST	O	00254	Filler Field 2 +	
22	26	TS	C	00255	Results Rpt/Status Chg - Date/Time+	
23	40	CM	O	00256	Charge to Practice +	
24	10	ID	O	00257	Diagnostic Serv Sect ID	Needed
25	1	ID	C	00258	Result Status +	Use F for final
26	400	CM	O	00259	Parent Result +	
27	200	TQ	O	00221	Quantity/Timing	
28	150	XCN	O	00260	Result Copies To	
29	150	CM	O	00261	Parent *	
30	20	ID	O	00262	Transportation Mode	
31	300	CE	O	00263	Reason for Study	Can store the ICD9 code for reimbursement
32	200	CM	O	00264	Principal Result Interpreter +	Needed

Appendix F: Message: Questions and Answers

33	200	CM	O	00265	Assistant Result Interpreter +	
34	200	CM	O	00266	Technician +	
35	200	CM	O	00267	Transcriptionist +	
36	26	TS	O	00268	Scheduled Date/Time +	
37	4	NM	O	01028	Number of Sample Containers *	
38	60	CE	O	01029	Transport Logistics of Collected Sample *	
39	200	CE	O	01030	Collector's Comment *	
40	60	CE	O	01031	Transport Arrangement Responsibility	
41	30	ID	O	01032	Transport Arranged	
42	1	ID	O	01033	Escort Required	
43	200	CE	O	01034	Planned Patient Transport Comment	

[Reporting Pathology Protocols (RPP) Messaging Work Group on October 29, 2003]

6 - Question: Should we use the CWE data type?

Discussion: The CWE data type was created for segments with both coded and text data. The CE data type in conjunction with String data could provide the same information. In the colon-rectum checklist, the CWE data type would only be used 3 – 4 times. For example RPP Item Number 13, Histologic Grade (hi/low) would be a place to use the CWE data type. A CWE data type would tell the receiving software to look for a code in text format. In general, text data should be used with the appropriate LOINC code, 22638-1 (see RPP Item Number 33, Additional Text on CAP checklist.)

Decision: We will use the CWE data type, but California and Cerner will employ different interpretations. Cerner will use the CWE only if the other answer is available.

[Reporting Pathology Protocols (RPP) Messaging Work Group on December 4, 2003]

7 - Question: When will the string (ST) data type be used and when will the text (TX) data type be used?

Discussion: Per HL7 and some CDC-NPCR HL7 implementation guidelines, the ST data type should be used for relatively short and left justified text while the TX data type should be used for longer text strings. If some text is not left justified, there could be data with leading blanks which could lead to special edits for those receiving the message. Another option for text is the FT data type which is used for special formatting commands to be embedded in long text strings.

Decision: We will use the ST data type for text less than 200 characters and the TX data type for text greater than or equal to 200 characters. Typically, the RPP Data Item Number 31, other polyps – text, would use the ST data type while the RPP Data Item Number 33, Additional Text on CAP checklist, would use the TX data type. This topic will be raised with the larger RPP team at the December 18, 2003 meeting.

[Reporting Pathology Protocols (RPP) Messaging Work Group on December 4, 2003]

8 - Question: The text question and answer names in the segments on the California sample message varies from those on the Cerner sample message. Should the text question/answer

Appendix F: Message: Questions and Answers

names be the same in the California message as those in the California message? Are the standardized LOINC names for informational purposes or are they fixed?

Discussion: The LOINC code defines the actual question and not the associated text. The purpose of the text is to make the message easier for humans to read.

Decision: The codes will be used to de-code the question and the answers, the associated text descriptions will be up to the local user. The text description could be a backup if the code is in error.

[Reporting Pathology Protocols (RPP) Messaging Work Group on December 4, 2003]

9 - Question: In the PV1 segment, how will the information for Sequence number 19, Visit Number, be obtained?

Discussion: In the Cerner system, this information is obtained via an interface with the ADT message.

Decision: This information will be optional, but will be sent if the corresponding administrative information is available.

[Reporting Pathology Protocols (RPP) Messaging Work Group on December 4, 2003]

10 - Question: Where should the ordering facility (or physician office) information is located in the message?

Discussion: Per HL7 this information should be located in the ORC message as follows: ORC-21, Ordering Facility Name; ORC-22, Ordering Facility Address; ORC-23, Ordering Facility Phone Number; and ORC-24, Ordering Provider Address. See the ORC attributes table.

Decision: We will use the above ORC segments. Linda Coles noted that, in the future, we may need to add some codes.

[Reporting Pathology Protocols (RPP) Messaging Work Group on December 4, 2003]

11 - Question: Where should information on the pathologists be located in the message?

Discussion: Cerner is currently using OBR-32, Principle Results Interpreter, with an interface code for the local pathologists code and, if available, the UPIN codes. Typically, UPIN codes are not available for pathologists.

Decision: Information on the pathologist should be located in OBR-32, Principle Results Interpreter, as a required field. Pathologist code rules for this Project should remain flexible.

[Reporting Pathology Protocols (RPP) on December 18, 2003]

12 - Question: Should the message contain a code to indicate a CAP cancer protocols synoptic checklist?

Decision: We will use OBR 44, procedure code, with the CAP checklist Name/Codes.   We will use the OBR 4, Universal Service ID, with a General code of 'Surgical Biopsy'.

[Reporting Pathology Protocols (RPP) Messaging Work Group on October 1, 2003]

Edited Addendum July 2004: "Checklist identifiers" were added to the January 2004 release of SNOMED to identify each checklist. Their Fully specified names in SNOMED begin with "College of American Pathologists Cancer Checklist..." It was decided to use these identifiers to indicate the checklist. This is also addressed in the "Discussion Addendum" for Question 13.

13 - Question: How should the message identify which checklist is used?

Appendix F: Message: Questions and Answers

Discussion: The procedure code could be used in OBR 44, but other checklists are not clearly related to the associate procedure code. Using OBR 4, universal service ID, with the source of specimen code or the surgical procedure code was discussed. This may be problematic i.e. cytology and smears. Using OBR 15, specimen source, was discussed. While this would work for colon-rectum checklist, it would probably not work for other sites.
Decision: No consensus. This question will remain on the agenda.

[Reporting Pathology Protocols (RPP) Messaging Work Group on October 29, 2003]

Discussion Addendum: There was a discussion about the specimen source. SNOMED has recently introduced a concept to indicate which CAP Checklist is in use. For example, in the Colon and Rectum Protocol there is a concept code for the Colon and Rectum Polypectomy checklist, the Rectum Local Excision checklist, and the Colon and Rectum Resection checklist. This addition will be reflected in the January 2004 version of the CAP Cancer Protocols and Checklists. Dr. van Berkum will share a draft version with the RPP team. Dr. van Berkum noted that the purple font narrative refers to editorial enhancements by SNOMED usually to clarify style discrepancies among the checklists.

[Reporting Pathology Protocols (RPP) on December 18, 2003]

14 - Question: Where should the Checklist Identifier code be placed in the HL7 message?
Discussion: While the Checklist Identifier is not a procedure per say, OBR-44 Procedure Code is a good candidate. We could bend the meaning of the Procedure Code and use for the Checklist Identifier. We will need to make this notation in the RPP implementation guide.
Decision: The Checklist Identifier code will be placed in OBR-44, Procedure Code. The corresponding coding system code will be SM, SNOMED.
[Reporting Pathology Protocols (RPP) Messaging Work Group on January 7, 2004]

15 - Question: If these new CAP Checklist identifier concepts are the answer codes, then what is the corresponding question code?
Discussion: SNOMED and/or LOINC should add such codes or HL7 may already contain a concept to handle this situation and a question code is therefore immaterial.
[Reporting Pathology Protocols (RPP) on December 18, 2003]

16 - Question: Which, if any, of the ORC Ordering Facility fields will be required?
Discussion: The Ordering Facility Name (ORC-21) will be required. In terms of facility coding systems, there are several options including the AHA schema and the CoC schema. We cannot mandate a specific coding system, but the message will so indicate.
Decision: Of these fields only the Ordering Facility Name (ORC-21) will be required.
[Reporting Pathology Protocols (RPP) Messaging Work Group on January 7, 2004]

17 - Question: Which administratively related data items will be required?
Discussion: Dr. Barry Gordon has and will distribute an Excel sheet which identifies these data items. Messaging Work Group members will go through this list and indicate which data items should be required. At a future Messaging Work Group meeting these lists will be reconciled, as much as possible, and then presented to the larger RPP Team. As part of HL7 some of these data items are required.

Appendix F: Message: Questions and Answers

Decision:
[Reporting Pathology Protocols (RPP) Messaging Work Group on January 7, 2004]

18 - Question: Should we use the January 2004 version of the Colon and Rectum Checklist?
This version has yet to be release, but discussion centered around the pre-release version
distributed on December 19, 2003.
Discussion: We won't know some of the codes until the final version are released in January
2004. This Checklist simplifies some of the concepts. For example, the lateral margin and
mucosal margin concepts have been combined into the mucosal/lateral margin concept. This
change is noted in the OBX Excel table. We want to use the latest version of the Checklist
unless the RPP implementation is slowed down.
Decision: We will use the January 2004 version of the Checklist but make adjustments so that
the implementation can proceed within the next 2 – 3 weeks.
[Reporting Pathology Protocols (RPP) Messaging Work Group on January 7, 2004]

19 - Question: Some of the new concepts in the January 2004 Checklist do not have associated
LOINC codes.
Discussion:
Decision: We will continue to search for the LOINC question code in the available LOINC
vocabulary and will request a code from the LOINC Board if one is not available. If LOINC
question codes are not available for any new concepts, we will use the SNOMED question code
and, if needed, local codes.
[Reporting Pathology Protocols (RPP) Messaging Work Group on January 7, 2004]

Appendix F: Message: Questions and Answers

Unresolved

1 - Question: How should the Project handle addendums (or updates) to the message?
Discussion: CoPath sends updates on a frequent basis with the original OBR segment and Addenda information in an additional OBR followed by OBX segments. The question of updates may be outside the scope of this project and may need to be handled manually.
[Reporting Pathology Protocols (RPP) Messaging Work Group on October 1, 2003]

2 - Question: Should there be multiple checklists for a specimen?
Discussion: We need some use case examples. These situations where a single specimen produces multiple cancer diagnoses should be rare. For the purposes of this Project, we should probably assume a single report produces a single checklist.
[Reporting Pathology Protocols (RPP) Messaging Work Group on October 1, 2003]

Checklist

1 - Question: Given that the CAP checklist SNOMED codes contain both the question and the answer, what is the utility of LOINC in the message?
Discussion: The LOINC codes are part of the CDC-NPCR laboratory implementation guide. Approximately, two years ago representatives from the RPP group approached LOINC to obtain question values for this Project. RPP was originally designed to use SNOMED as the answer value and LOINC as the question value. The message could contain both the LOINC question value and the SNOMED question value. Co-Path has never used the LOINC codes.
[Reporting Pathology Protocols (RPP) Messaging Work Group on October 1, 2003]

2 - Question: What do we do with items that are not coded such as the "Other (specify) _____" items, and the comment at the end? How should free text be handled?
Discussion: A related question – should this project also send the final diagnosis and clinical history as text? The inclusion of clinical history is outside the scope of this project and as such will be left out. We should follow the CAP cancer protocols, but we have the option to add at a later date. Cerner is currently sending text as a separate OBX. There is a separate NAACCR committee addressing the issue of submitting text in pathology reports.
Decision: Use the LOINC question code as specified in the "OBX results Questions with proposed SNOMED and LOINC codes for colorectal checklist" Excel file spreadsheet. As examples see the RPP Item Numbers 13, Histologic Grade (hi/low), and 33, Additional Text on CAP checklist.
[Reporting Pathology Protocols (RPP) Messaging Work Group on October 29, 2003]

3 - Question: Many line items require that user fill in a response (usually a number). These line items also have associated SNOMED CT codes. But in HL7 the "answer" is either a coded value or a numeric value, not both. How should we handle these (numerous) cases? For example, on the Local Excision checklist the first section is Specimen Integrity, which is assigned a SNOMED code R-100A8. Under this there's an item for "Number of pieces" that requires that a numeric value, and that has an associated code F-048D8 "Number of pieces in fragmented specimen."
Discussion: The LOINC group hated this concept when it was presented for this project. Sending redundant information in the message is acceptable. In future iterations of this

Appendix F: Message: Questions and Answers

checklist, the CAP will add another question for Specimen Integrity, "not specified." This type of situation also exists with the tumor size and the associated additional dimensions questions.
Decision: The screen should look like the CAP cancer protocol checklist and, as such, there should be two fields with an OBX for each in this type of situation. See RPP Item Number 34, Number of Pieces.
[Reporting Pathology Protocols (RPP) Messaging Work Group on October 29, 2003]

4 - Question: On Local Excision, under Tumor Site, TWO codes are listed, and a note says that the two are required. The first item in this section asks for a distance in cm. If we adopt the rule suggested above, the two codes associated with Tumor Site will be ignored, and we'll send the one from the specimen line item instead (R-00266 Distance from anal verge). However, it is not clear what to send if the second item in the section is selected. Instead of the usual "question" code, we have 2 codes. And this is further complicated by a note that says that the "question" code really should be R-00266, which is neither of the 2 codes listed for the section.
Discussion: Tumor Site in the Polypectomy and Resection checklists has a number of sub-sites (i.e. cecum, right (ascending) colon, etc.), while the corresponding information in Local Excision (rectum) has an implied site of rectum.
Decision: The rectum site code should automatically be sent for Local Excision, Tumor Site. One answer should be sent of each question. See RPP Item Number 35, Distance from Anal Verge, and 36, Distance from Anal Verge unknown.
[Reporting Pathology Protocols (RPP) Messaging Work Group on October 29, 2003]

Discussion Addendum: I'd like to respond again to the questions regarding this section. I have included the section and its SNOMED codes below:

*TUMOR SITE [R-0025A, 371480007] Tumor site (observable entity) [T-59600, 34402009] Rectum structure (body structure) Will require two codes to capture tumor site implied in checklist title
*Distance from anal verge (per clinical report): ___ cm [R-00266, 371490004] Distance of tumor from anal verge (observable entity)
*___ Distance from anal verge unknown [R-0027C, 372298005] Distance of tumor from anal verge unknown (finding) this answers [R-00266, 371490004] Distance of tumor from anal verge (observable entity) if there is not a numerical answer that can be provided.

Most items on the checklist are treated in a "question" and "answer" format. The header is usually the question and the answer is usually one of the choices offered below it. However, the checklists had multiple authors and while their formats are generally consistent, they are not always consistent. I have tried to accommodate for some of those inconsistencies.

For the section shown above, the majority of the checklists offer anatomic choices for the site of origin of the tumor under "TUMOR SITE". On this checklist, since the checklist applies only to "Rectum: Local excision" the site of rectum is implied in the checklist title. However, I was not sure how different vendors would capture that information, so I offered the SNOMED code for "Rectum structure" paired with the header "Tumor site" as if it was the only answer or choice under "Tumor site".

Appendix F: Message: Questions and Answers

On this checklist, the author has actually offered other choices under "Tumor site" than the anatomic choices usually offered on other checklists. What the author has really done is added a different question (or a sub-header) under "Tumor site". The pathologist is not really being asked the anatomic "Tumor site" but rather to identify where the tumor is in relation to the anal verge. The way we intend for this to be coded is that if the pathologist answers the distance in cm with a numerical value, then that numerical value will answer: [R-00266, 371490004] Distance of tumor from anal verge (observable entity). If they chose "___ Distance of tumor from anal verge unknown" then "[R-0027C, 372298005] Distance of tumor from anal verge unknown (finding) " will answer: [R-00266, 371490004] Distance of tumor from anal verge (observable entity).

In your draft, the following statement (referring to the section shown above) is made: "And this is further complicated by a note that says that the "question" code really should be R-00266, which is neither of the 2 codes listed for the section." My explanation above is why I included a note clarifying which "question" code should be paired with this "answer" code.

There are quite a few instances in the checklists where there are "sub-questions" or (sub-headers) under the "questions" (or headers). In most cases, we are relying on the implementer to ascertain from the text that the items nested under a sub-header are usually answering the sub-header.

Another example of this is shown below in an excerpt from the Margins section of the same checklist (Rectum: Local excision):

MARGINS (check all that apply) [R-00472, 395535007] Status of surgical margin involvement by tumor (observable entity) ___ Margins cannot be assessed [R-00474, 395537004] Surgical margin involvement by tumor cannot be assessed (finding) Lateral margin [R-00437, 384786009] Status of surgical lateral (mucosal/mural) margin involvement by tumor (observable entity) ___ Uninvolved by invasive carcinoma [R-0045E, 384804002] Surgical lateral (mucosal/mural) margin uninvolved by malignant neoplasm (finding)

For this section, "___ Margins cannot be assessed" is the answer to "[R-00472, 395535007] Status of surgical margin involvement by tumor (observable entity)". However, "___ Uninvolved by invasive carcinoma" is not the answer to "[R-00472, 395535007] Status of surgical margin involvement by tumor (observable entity)". Instead, "___ Uninvolved by invasive carcinoma" answers the "sub-header" of "Lateral Margin". Thus, [R-0045E, 384804002] Surgical lateral (mucosal/mural) margin uninvolved by malignant neoplasm (finding) answers [R-00437, 384786009] Status of surgical lateral (mucosal/mural) margin involvement by tumor (observable entity) not [R-00472, 395535007] Status of surgical margin involvement by tumor (observable entity). This is why I have actually added the words "lateral margin" into the concepts fully specified names. We are not saying that all margins are uninvolved by invasive carcinoma. We are specifying that only the "lateral margin" is uninvolved by invasive carcinoma.

[Reporting Pathology Protocols (RPP) Messaging Work Group on October 29, 2003 - Addendum]

5 - Question: At the top of each checklist there are a few codes for the following: procedure, specimen type (observable entity) and specimen obtained from. Will these types of codes exist for other sites, in addition to colon-rectum?

Appendix F: Message: Questions and Answers

Decision: Reporting Pathology Protocols (RPP) Messaging Work Group on October 29, 2003]

Discussion Addendum: Sometimes. The "Specimen type" or "Tumor site" codes will appear at the top of other checklists when the information pertaining to "Specimen type" or "Tumor site" is not captured in the content of the actual checklist but rather implied in the checklist title (as it was for the Rectum checklist where the only possible tumor site was rectum). For most checklist titles, if the "procedure" could be captured by a single SNOMED concept, it was given a code. For example, for "Rectum: Local excision", the code [P1-5832A, 287784004] Local excision of rectum (procedure) was appropriate. However, for some checklists, such as the breast checklist, where the title was "BREAST: Excision Less Than Total Mastectomy (Includes Wire-Guided Localization Excisions); Total Mastectomy, Modified Radical Mastectomy, Radical Mastectomy ", no single procedure code in SNOMED exists to capture this.

Thus, there is not one type of code (Specimen type, Tumor Site, or Procedure) that can be relied upon to always be at the top of each checklist that could be used to identify that checklist. This was addressed through the creation of "Checklist identifiers" in SNOMED to identify each checklist. (See Question 12 under HL7 message.)

[Reporting Pathology Protocols (RPP) Messaging Work Group on October 29, 2003 - Addendum]

6 - Question: When I originally posed this question, I regret that I selected the Specimen Integrity area as my example. Specimen Integrity brings up other questions that I had not intended to ask. Let's just look at Tumor Size, and Greatest Dimension, instead. The "question" based upon the heading is F-02BBE Tumor size (observable entity). The "answer" is R-00272 Tumor size, largest dimension (observable entity). Wait, no, that's not the answer; the answer is a numeric value for a number of cm. What I propose to do in this situation is to send R-00272 as the "question code" (or I guess it's supposed to be the LOINC equivalent of this SNOMED code), send the numeric value as the "answer", and ignore F-02BBE altogether as it doesn't add any additional information.
Answer: Yes. It makes sense. "Tumor size largest dimension" was never intended to be the answer. It does not have a check box in front of it that the user can check. Instead, it was a sub header under tumor size. The concept R-00272 Tumor size, largest dimension (observable entity) as a question combined with the numerical value 2 cm will in essence constitute a "finding" of "Largest dimension of tumor is 2 cm." An additional note here is that any SNOMED concept from the "Observable entity" hierarchy is never intended as an answer. A concept with the "Observable entity" tag such as Tumor size (observable entity) are intended as metadata (questions) to be answered by selecting from one of the checkable items below it by the insertion of a numerical or written answer.
[Reporting Pathology Protocols (RPP) Summary of November 13, 2003 - E-mails Between Monique van Berkum and Zeke Holland]

7 - Question: Can this be generalized to all items where the user has to fill in a value? It seems to work for the several cases I have looked at, but I'm reluctant to draw a conclusion about this. It worries me that we have codes associated with headings that we would ignore. But if this works, it works. It's important (to me, at least) that we come up with generic ways to deal with

Appendix F: Message: Questions and Answers

these constructs. We software developers will not be happy if we have to write special logic for individual items!

Answer: Without looking at all 42 checklists, I am not 100% sure that this can be generalized to all items where the user has to fill in a value but I suspect it could be. There are going to be many cases where the header will be ignored for some but not all items below it.

For the example shown below, "Greatest dimension: ___ cm" does not have a checkbox in front of it that can be checked. It is not an answer to "Polyp size", but rather, a "sub question" that will require an answer. In contrast, "___ cannot be determined" has a checkbox in front of it. It is an answer to "Polyp size" and in that case the header of "Polyp size" should not be ignored.

Polyp size
Greatest dimension: ___ cm
*Additional dimensions: ___ x ___ cm
___ cannot be determined
[Reporting Pathology Protocols (RPP) Summary of November 13, 2003 - E-mails Between Monique van Berkum and Zeke Holland]

8 - Questions: Based upon Dr. van Berkum's comments, can't the two codes associated with the heading -- R-0025A Tumor site (observable entity) and T-59600 Rectum structure (body structure) be "paired codes" that are always associated with the checklist, rather than being specifically associated with Tumor Site?

Then the Tumor Site "question" code would be R-00266 Distance of tumor from anal verge, and the first possible "answer" would be the numeric value, and the second possible answer would be the coded value R-0027C Distance of tumor from anal verge unknown (finding).

Answer: The code "R-0025A Tumor site (observable entity)" and the concept I paired with it "T-59600 Rectum structure (body structure)" was my way of compensating for the fact that the format of each checklist is not always consistent. When the authors started on the checklist they were thinking of them as tools for the pathologist and not necessarily as documents that would be coded electronically. SNOMED entered the picture later in the game. We are gradually influencing the cancer committee to be even more consistent in their style.
[Reporting Pathology Protocols (RPP) Summary of November 13, 2003 - E-mails Between Monique van Berkum and Zeke Holland]

9 - Question: You asked: "Can't the two codes associated with the heading -- R-0025A Tumor site (observable entity) and T-59600 Rectum structure (body structure) is "paired codes" that are always associated with the checklist, rather than being specifically associated with Tumor Site?"
Answer: No. That approach may work for this one checklist but it won't work for all checklists. Some checklists offer 10 sites under Tumor Site. Which one would you chose to "always" associate with the checklist?
[Reporting Pathology Protocols (RPP) Summary of November 13, 2003 - E-mails Between Monique van Berkum and Zeke Holland]

10 – Question: You stated: "Then the Tumor Site "question" code would be R-00266 Distance of tumor from anal verge, and the first possible "answer" would be the numeric value, and the

second possible answer would be the coded value R-0027C Distance of tumor from anal verge unknown (finding)."

Answer: You are right with respect to what the two answer choices for R-00266 Distance of tumor from anal verge would be. However, the Tumor Site "question" code would not be R-00266 Distance of tumor from anal verge, The "Distance of tumor from anal verge____" question code would be R-00266 Distance of tumor from anal verge. The Tumor Site "question" code will still be R-0025A Tumor site (observable entity).

[Reporting Pathology Protocols (RPP) Summary of November 13, 2003 - E-mails Between Monique van Berkum and Zeke Holland]

11 - Question: In the Colon and Rectum checklist on page 14 in the Mesorectum section (optional), there is not an option for an invasion. How should situations where no invasion occurs be handled?

Discussion: Receivers of data would like to know "no invasion" as opposed to "we didn't bother to send this optional item." Mary will discuss with Dr. Compton.

[Reporting Pathology Protocols (RPP) on November 20, 2003]

Edited Addendum July 2004: It turns out that this section was not referring to involvement of the mesorectum by tumor but rather to intactness of the mesorectal specimen. Therefore, the header will be changed (in the January 2005 release of the uncoded checklists) to "Intactness of Mesorectum" and the codes I had supplied for this section did not capture the meaning of the section and needed to be replaced. The new codes were shared with the RPP group in an e-mail sent 4/12/2004 and are included as Appendix B in this Report.

12 - Question: The "Mesorectum" section under the Colon and Rectum Resection on page 14 does not contain the option of none. How should we handle this situation?

Discussion: This is more a problem with the CAP cancer protocols checklists which are not always consistent especially in the optional data items. This will be reviewed at future Cancer Protocols – SNOMED meetings.

Decision: For the purpose of RPP, we will use the checklist as it exists today. If the answer to the Mesorectum (G-F7B9) question is none, no corresponding information will be sent.

[Reporting Pathology Protocols (RPP) Messaging Work Group on December 4, 2003]

Edited Addendum July 2004: This is actually the same question as Question 11 above. The same answer applies:

It turns out that this section was not referring to involvement of the mesorectum by tumor but rather to intactness of the mesorectal specimen. Therefore, the header will be changed (in the January 2005 release of the uncoded checklists) to "Intactness of Mesorectum" and the codes I had supplied for this section did not capture the meaning of the section and needed to be replaced. The new codes were shared with the RPP group in an e-mail sent 4/12/2004 and are included as Appendix B in this Report.

13 - Question: Where in the message should the ordering facility or the physician address be recorded?

Discussion: A later draft version of 2.3.1 does contain OBR attributes related to the ordering facility. To be investigated and resolved.

Appendix F: Message: Questions and Answers

[Reporting Pathology Protocols (RPP) on November 20, 2003]

<u>14 - Question</u>: The "Margins" section under the Colon and Rectum Resection on page 17 has a sub-headings titled "Distance of tumor from closest margin: ____" and "Specify margin" which could refer to either the proximal, distal, or circumferential margins.
<u>Discussion</u>:
<u>Decision</u>: We will make these questions optional and answer only if all margins were uninvolved and only if appropriate.
[Reporting Pathology Protocols (RPP) Messaging Work Group on December 4, 2003]

Additionally this was presented at the March 2004 meeting of the Cancer Committee and the wording for this section will change slightly for clarification purposes in January 2005. Also, in the July 2004 RPP call Dr. Barry Gordon raised the issue that it would be nice to have SNOMED codes for the margin choices which are possible answers to "Specify margin". I will investigate this with Dr. Spackman.

<u>15 - Question</u>: In the Resection section under Mesenteric margin, the concept "Distance of invasive carcinoma from closest margin" on page 19 gives two units of measures: mm and cm. This could create some problems with the front end implementation. Which should unit of measure should we use?
<u>Discussion</u>:
<u>Decision</u>: For RPP, messages the standard unit of measure will be mm. For the present in this project, software developers will continue to use mm as the standard unit of measure for the front end of the system.
[Reporting Pathology Protocols (RPP) Messaging Work Group on January 7, 2004]

<u>16 - Question</u>: The January 2004 Checklist contains some new concepts including "Specimen Integrity", "Tumor Size Cannot be Determined", "Type of Polyp", and "Mesenteric Margin".
<u>Discussion</u>: Dr. Barry Gordon has incorporated these concepts into the OBX Excel table. Some of these concepts lack both SNOMED and LOINC codes, but the SNOMED codes should be available with the January 2004 version (vs. the pre-release version). In the OBX Excel table for the next meeting, Dr. Gordon will search for appropriate LOINC codes. If none are available we will use the SNOMED question code, if available, or a local code.
<u>Decision</u>:
[Reporting Pathology Protocols (RPP) Messaging Work Group on January 7, 2004]

<u>17 - Question</u>: Which SNOMED CT codes should be used for RPP, the shorter or the longer?
<u>Discussion</u>: Both are unique identifiers for the concept, but the longer codes contain more information. The longer numeric code, referred to as the ConceptID, is the code recommended for use by SNOMED CT.
<u>Decision</u>: We will use the longer codes.
[Reporting Pathology Protocols (RPP) Messaging Work Group on January 7, 2004]

<u>18 - Question</u>: How should the Specimen Type and Specimen paired codes at the beginning of the Polypectomy and Local Excision Checklists is handled?
<u>Discussion</u>:

Appendix F: Message: Questions and Answers

Decision: For the Local Excision (page 8), the Specimen Type of "Specimen from rectum obtained by transanal disk excision" the SNOMED code of 122653009 should be sent in the RPP-1 field (see Excel table), identified by the LOINC code of 33722-0. A similar coding for polypectomy should occur.
[Reporting Pathology Protocols (RPP) Messaging Work Group on January 7, 2004]

19 - Question: On page 8 under the Local Excision Checklist, should the Tumor Site and Rectum structure paired codes be handled in the same way (See 10 – Question)?
Discussion: The Tumor Site codes do not answer the Tumor Site question, but rather another question. Because Rectum is the only body structure code for this Checklist, the Rectum body structure code is implied. The line items under Tumor Site do not answer the type of questions routinely asked under this header on other checklists. Normally, under Tumor Site, the choices given are body sites. In this case, the line items under Tumor Site such as "Distance of tumor from anal verge" are actually asking other questions. Because the site that is implied by the title of this section is Rectum, Dr. van Berkum (SNOMED) has provided the code for Rectum and paired it with the code for Tumor site.
Decision: The Tumor Site code and the Body Structure code will be included in one OBX segment. For Local Excision (page 8), the SNOMED code of 34402009 for rectum body structure goes into RPP-4 (see Excel table) in an OBX.
[Reporting Pathology Protocols (RPP) Messaging Work Group on January 7, 2004]

20 - Question: On page 11 of the Local Excision Checklist, how should "Distance of invasive carcinoma from…" be coded if the margin is involved?
Discussion:
Decision: If "Uninvolved by invasive carcinoma" is not checked then the questions "Distance of invasive carcinoma from …." and "*Specify location (e.g., o'clock position), if possible:" cannot be answered. If "Uninvolved by invasive carcinoma" is checked, then "Distance of invasive carcinoma from …." seems to become a mandatory item whereas "*Specify location (e.g., o'clock position), if possible:" would still be optional.
[Reporting Pathology Protocols (RPP) Messaging Work Group on January 7, 2004]

21 - Question: For the Local Excision Checklist (page 11), why is "Distance of invasive carcinoma from closest lateral margin" under Lateral Margin worded differently from the "Distance of invasive carcinoma from margin" under Deep Margin?
Discussion: There can be more than one lateral margin on a specimen (e.g. left lateral margin or a right lateral margin) but there is only one deep margin. That is why the word "closest" was added to the phrase. And, when they enter the distance of the tumor from the closest lateral margin, they are then given the option of specifying which lateral margin they are referring to.
Decision:
[Reporting Pathology Protocols (RPP) Messaging Work Group on January 7, 2004]

22 - Question: How is the "Distance of invasive carcinoma from closest lateral margin" concept in the Local Excision Checklist (page 11) different from the "Distance of tumor from closest margin" (RPP-23 in Excel table)?
Discussion: The margins section of the Cancer checklists makes distinctions between Carcinoma in situ, invasive carcinoma, and tumor. In this section of the checklist, in general, "tumor" could be used to mean either "in situ" or "invasive carcinoma". In coding concepts for the "Margins"

Appendix F: Message: Questions and Answers

section, SNOMED has tried to use the words "Malignant neoplasm" where the cancer committee uses "invasive carcinoma". For this reason, a literal item on the checklist like "Distance of invasive carcinoma from margin" is coded with Distance of malignant neoplasm from margin (observable entity) not "Distance of tumor from margin (observable entity)". Even when not using SNOMED concepts, I (Dr. van Berkum) would caution against substituting the word tumor for invasive carcinoma in this section of the checklist.

<u>Decision</u>:

[Reporting Pathology Protocols (RPP) Messaging Work Group on January 7, 2004]

<u>23 - Question</u>: How is "Distance of invasive carcinoma from closest lateral margin" in the Local Excision Checklist (page 11) different from the "Distance of invasive carcinoma from closest margin" in the Resection Checklist (page 19)?

<u>Discussion</u>:   The different way in which the "Distance of invasive carcinoma from closest margin" question was handled on page 19 may be because, for this section, this information only has prognostic significance when all margins are uninvolved. However, the way it is handled on page 19 may create problems since "Distance of invasive carcinoma from closest margin:" and "Specify margin:" are not asterisked items. However, it seems they can only be filled in if all the margins above them are uninvolved by tumor. These types of items are tricky because they are only mandatory in a particular circumstance. I (Dr. van Berkum) will suggest at the committee meeting in March that this section be reworded in some way (see below).

"If all the above margins are uninvolved by tumor then provide:

   Distance of invasive carcinoma from closest margin:

   Specify margin: _____ "

<u>Decision</u>:

[Reporting Pathology Protocols (RPP) Messaging Work Group on January 7, 2004]

<u>Edited Addendum July 2004</u>: This seems to have been accepted at the March meeting and should appear in the January 2005 edition posted by the CAP.

Appendix F: Message: Questions and Answers

Appendix G: Local Excision (Transanal Disk Excision) Checklist by Required and Non-Required Status

Required Data Elements (*N* = 12):
- Specimen integrity
- Tumor size
- Histologic type
- Histologic grade
- Primary tumor
- Regional lymph nodes
- Specify, examined (regional lymph nodes)
- Specify, involved (regional lymph nodes)
- Margins (lateral and deep)
- Lymphatic invasion
- Venous invasion

Nonrequired Data Elements (*N* = 14):
- Number of pieces (specimen integrity)
- Tumor site
- Tumor configuration
- Additional dimensions (tumor size)
- pT3 a/b and pT3 c/d
- Specify location (lateral margin – uninvolved and involved)
- Involved by carcinoma in situ/adenoma (lateral margin)
- Intramural/extramural (lymphatic invasion)
- Intramural/extramural (venous invasion)
- Perineural invasion
- Tumor border configuration
- Intratumoral/peritumoral lymphocytic response
- Additional pathologic findings

Appendix H: Resection Checklist by Required and Non-Required Status

Required Data Elements (*N* = 17):
- Specimen type
- Tumor site
- Tumor size
- Histologic type
- Histologic grade
- Primary tumor
- Regional lymph nodes
- Specify, examined (regional lymph nodes)
- Specify, involved (regional lymph nodes)
- Distant metastasis
- Margin, proximal
- Margin, distal
- Margin, radial
- Distance of tumor from closest margin
- Specify margin
- Lymphatic invasion
- Venous invasion

Non-required Data Elements (*N* = 13):
- Length (specimen type)
- Tumor configuration
- Additional dimensions (tumor size)
- Mesorectum
- PT3 a/b/ or pT3 c/d
- Specify site (distant metastasis)
- Intramural/extramural (lymphatic invasion)
- Intramural/extramural (venous invasion)
- Perineural invasion
- Tumor border configuration
- Intratumoral/peritumoral lymphocytic response
- Additional pathologic findings

Appendix I: SEER Extent of Disease Schemes of Regional Lymph Node Involvement for Colorectal Cancers

COLON (incl. Flexures and Appendix)
ICD-O-3 Topography Range: C18.0-C18.9

LYMPH NODES
0   No lymph node involvement
- - - - - - - - - - - - - - - - -
REGIONAL Lymph Nodes
1   **All colon subsites**:
       Epicolic (adjacent to bowel wall)
       Paracolic/pericolic
       Colic, NOS
       Nodule(s) in pericolic fat
2   **Cecum and Appendix**:
       Cecal: anterior, posterior, NOS
       Ileocolic
       Right colic
       Ascending colon:
       Ileocolic
       Right colic
       Middle colic
    Transverse colon and flexures:
       Middle colic
       Right colic for **hepatic flexure only**
       Left colic for **splenic flexure only**
       Inferior mesenteric for **splenic**
       flexure only
    Descending colon:
       Left colic
       Sigmoid
       Inferior mesenteric
    Sigmoid:
       Sigmoidal (sigmoid mesenteric)
       Superior hemorrhoidal
       Superior rectal
       Inferior mesenteric
3   Mesenteric, NOS
       Regional lymph node(s), NOS
- - - - - - - - - - - - - - - - -
DISTANT Lymph Nodes
7   Other than above, incl. superior mesenteric
- - - - - - - - - - - - - - - - -
8   Lymph Nodes, NOS
9   UNKNOWN; not stated

RECTOSIGMOID, RECTUM
ICD-O-3 Topography Range: C19.9, C20.9

LYMPH NODES
0   No lymph node involvement

- - - - - - - - - - - - - - - - -

REGIONAL Lymph Nodes
1 Rectosigmoid:
> Paracolic/pericolic
> Perirectal
> Nodule(s) in pericolic fat

 Rectum:
> Perirectal
> Nodule(s) in perirectal fat

2 Rectosigmoid:
> Hemorrhoidal, superior or middle
> Left colic (incl. colic, NOS)
> Superior rectal
> Sigmoidal (sigmoid mesenteric)
> Inferior mesenteric

 Rectum:
> Sigmoidal
> Sigmoid mesenteric
> Inferior mesenteric
> Hemorrhoidal, superior, middle or inferior |
> Sacral (lateral, presacral, sacral promontory
> {Gerota's}, or NOS)
> Internal iliac (hypogastric)

3 Mesenteric, NOS
> Regional lymph node(s), NOS

- - - - - - - - - - - - - - - - -

DISTANT Lymph Nodes
7 Other than above

- - - - - - - - - - - - - - - - -

8 Lymph Nodes, NOS
9 UNKNOWN; not stated

Appendix I: SEER EOD Schemes of Regional Lymph Node Involvement for Colorectal Cancers

Appendix J: California RPP Evaluation Measures

Reporting Pathology Protocols - College of Pathologists – Colon and Rectum Protocols - UCI Medical Center/California Cancer Registry, Assessments for Completeness, Timeliness, and Quality
April 23, 2003

1. **Completeness**

   a) **Does the checklist provide the necessary information to code the state-required extent of disease data items?**
      Process: Using the information on the CAP checklist, assign SEER extent of disease (EOD) codes. Using the narrative report (same tumor), assign SEER EOD codes. The SEER EOD data items are tumor size, extension, and lymph nodes.
      Analysis: Compare results.

   b) **Is the CAP reporting software sending all reports to the cancer registry?**
      Process: Compare the checklist reports received in the cancer registry with pathology reports gathered manually.
      Analysis: Calculate the percentage of missed checklist reports.

   c) **Was a checklist report completed for all applicable cases?**
      Process: Compare narrative pathology reports identified through routine case-finding procedures with all electronic checklist reports.
      Analysis: Calculate percentage of cases for which a checklist was not completed.

2. **Timeliness/Efficiency**

   a) **Does it take less time for the cancer registrar to abstract information from the CAP checklist as opposed to the narrative pathology report?**
      Process: Measure, in minutes, the time it takes to abstract certain data items from the narrative report and the CAP checklist (reports will be used for the same specimen). All narrative reports will be abstracted one day, and all checklist reports will be abstracted the next day. The same staff member will perform this activity. Data items to be abstracted are tumor size, number of lymph nodes examined, number of lymph nodes positive, histology, extent of invasion (EOD), and pathologic AJCC staging (T and N only), margins, lymphatic, venous, and perineural invasion.
      Analysis: Compare results.

   b) **Does it take less time for the pathologist to complete the CAP checklist as opposed to a narrative pathology report?**
      Process: The pathologist will complete both the CAP checklist and a narrative report for all colorectal cases. The time to complete each report will be measured. ****method of measuring to be determined****
      Analysis: Compare results.

3. QUALITY/ACCURACY

a) **Are the codes generated for certain data items from the CAP checklist as accurate as the codes produced by cancer registry staff?**

Process: Cancer registry staff will code site, histology, and AJCC staging (T and N only) for all narrative reports for a designated time period.

Analysis: Compare codes generated by the electronic CAP checklist with codes produced by the cancer registry staff. Identify problem areas.

b) **Does using the checklist format enhance the quality of the data?**

Process: Using narrative pathology reports from the previous year, complete a checklist for each report.

Analysis: Identify data items on the checklist that could not be completed by using the narrative report.

Appendix J: California RPP Evaluation Measures

Appendix K: Ohio RPP Evaluation Measures

Below are Ohio's evaluation measures.

Completeness/Quality:

1. Assessment of Quality, Completeness
   Dr. Willis, the participating pathologist from UHC, will enter data from selected narrative reports of colorectal malignancies into the new system. The narrative reports and the RPP checklist reports from the new system being developed by the project team will be sent to OCISS along with the codes for four data items from the checklist system. Three of these data items—site, histology, and stage—were selected for evaluation of completeness and quality because they are critical to the surveillance of cancer; i.e., they are necessary for the calculation of cancer rates in Ohio. Because cancer surveillance is the main purpose of the state's cancer registry, these were determined to be data items of interest for purposes of assessment for this project. In addition, grade was selected as a data item for evaluation because of its importance as a prognostic indicator and a determinant of treatment for use in the medical setting.

   Two OCISS certified registrars will code the four data items from each narrative pathology report. The two sets of codes will be compared to determine a "gold standard." Discrepancies will be resolved by a third, senior certified registrar.

   The OCISS "gold standard" codes will be entered into an Excel database along with the RPP checklist codes. Once all data are entered, completeness and accuracy will be determined. OCISS registrars will look at discrepancies to determine why they exist, whether it might be something wrong with the programming, something they might be miscoding, or something the pathologist may not agree with them about.

   It is noted here that, in practical use, the system under development assures that it will be the pathologist who determines what exact codes are assigned to each cancer case based on each pathologic analysis, rather than the cancer registrar reading a narrative report and interpreting from it.

   Completeness: The percent of blanks, overall and for each data item, among the RPP data, but not among the OCISS data.

   Quality: The percent of matches on a case-by-case basis between OCISS and RPP data items, overall and for each data item.

2. Physician assessment of quality of checklist
   Physicians will be asked to look at the checklist reports and comments on whether they would prefer them over current reports and whether they would save time. Questions appear on the UHC questionnaire.

3. Pathologists' assessment of quality of checklist
   UHC pathologists will be surveyed to determine what they think of the idea of using a checklist type system. Questions appear on the UHC questionnaire.

4. Reporting source registrars in some of Ohio's hospitals will be asked to help survey some of their physicians and pathologists to get an idea of how they might welcome standardized pathology reporting. This might provide some insight about the acceptance that standardization of pathology data might find in the medical community.

Timeliness:
1. Survey Pathology Staff and Cancer Registrars Entering Data:
Pathologist—Does the synoptic data entry system save time? Does it suffice to replace the dictated narrative report? Questions about saving time are to be included on surveys.

Cancer registrars will be asked to review pathology narrative reports and corresponding checklists—does the checklist report save time in transferring information to registry records? This will be done with OCISS registrars.

Attending physician—does interpreting the checklist report save time versus the narrative report? Does it contain sufficient information for the physician? Would the physician prefer receiving the checklist report instead of the narrative report?

RPP evaluation sheet, University Hospital of Cleveland: Completeness and Quality

For case number _____   Name_____   DDx_____

Item	OCISS Abstract	Checklist Report	'OK' if matched 'I' if incomplete
1 Site	_____	_____	_____
2 Histology	_____	_____	_____
3 Grade	_____	_____	_____
4 T/N Stage	_____	_____	_____
	M = Missing information	B = Blank, not incomplete	B on Checklist = I; however, M on Abstract and B on Checklist = OK

ANALYSES: At the end of a selected time period, the following analyses will be performed.

Completeness: Where the abstract column shows a value other than M and the checklist column shows a B (blank), mark I. Determine percent of reports with no "I"s for each item. This measures completeness of data for each item.

Quality: Determine the percent that matches for each data item.

Appendix K: Ohio RPP Evaluation Measures

Appendix L: Ohio RPP Physician and Pathologist Survey
Ohio Department of Health

Dear Cancer Incidence Reporting Source:

Thanks for offering to help us evaluate a new method for collecting pathology data on cancers for a project initiated and funded by the Centers for Disease Control's National Program of Cancer Registries in collaboration with the College of American Pathologists. This should not require a great deal of anyone's time, but will help us determine the usefulness of this project.

There are four parts to this:

(1) You review and comment on the sample Surgical Pathology Report we have enclosed and let us know what you think in the blank spaces below.

(2) Give the Surgical Pathology Report to a few of your physicians who diagnose and treat cancers. Then have them take a minute to look at the College of American Pathologists Tumor Summary and ask them to answer the few questions on the Survey Sheet for Physicians and write down the answers.

(3) Give the Colon and Rectum "Checklists" to one or more of your pathologists who analyze biopsy specimens for cancer to review briefly. Then ask them the questions on the Survey Sheet for Pathologists and write down the answers.

(4) Finally, please attach a <u>blank copy of a sample path report produced by this pathologist,</u> so the OCISS can get a better idea of what current practice is at your hospital.
Return by March 8, 2005 to:
Georgette G. Haydu, MA, Administrative Manager
Ohio Cancer Incidence Surveillance System
Ohio Department of Health | For more information contact: |
PO Box 118
Columbus, Ohio 43216-011   Phone: 614-466-5350
Email: ghaydu@odh ohio.gov

<u>Please fill in the following:</u>
 Reporting Source Contact Name_____
Hospital_____ American College of Surgeons Accredited? Y___ N___
OCISS Reporting Source Number_____ Phone _____

<u>Surgical Pathology Laboratory Report – cancer reporting source evaluation:</u>
Do you think it would save some time for you in your gathering of cancer data to have a Tumor Summary Section on pathology reports like the one at the beginning of this report: Y___ N ___ Don't Know____

<u>Please explain your answer:</u>

<u>Additional comments:</u>

RPP Physicians Survey
The Ohio Cancer Incidence Surveillance System
Ohio Department of Health

Hospital_____ **OCISS ID**_____ **Date**_____

Cancer Reporting Contact_____ **Phone** _____

Physician name_____

Give the Surgical Pathology Report to the physician and tell him/her:
- You have received a blanked out copy of a new type of Surgical Pathology Report now being developed under a grant from the National Program of Cancer Registries at the Centers for Disease Control. It is based on standardized coding of cancer pathology data. This one is for a colorectal cancer, but might be used for any type of cancer.

Read the following and record the physician's answers to questions:

- What types of cancer do you diagnose and/or treat?_____

- Please look at the Surgical Pathology Report that begins with **College of American Pathologists Tumor Summary**. Look at that section in particular. Would you prefer to receive this type of report from your pathology lab for colorectal and/or other types of cancers rather than the one you now receive?

- I would prefer this type of report. Check one:

Strongly Agree	Agree	Don't Know	Disagree	Strongly Disagree
_____	_____	_____	_____	_____

- Physician's Comments:

- This type of report might save time. Check one:

Strongly Agree	Agree	Don't Know	Disagree	Strongly Disagree
_____	_____	_____	_____	_____

- Comments

RPP Pathologist Survey
The Ohio Cancer Incidence Surveillance System
Ohio Department of Health

Hospital_____ **Date**_____

Cancer Reporting Contact_____ **Phone**_____

_____

Pathologist's name_____

Give the Checklist to the pathologist

Read this part to the pathologist:
You have received Checklists for recording data for colorectal biopsies by Polypectomy, Local Excision, Resection. These checklists might be <u>developed for any type of cancer</u> and this one, for a colorectal cancer, is just a sample for you evaluate. Please briefly look at these and rate your agreement with the following:

- I like the idea of standardizing pathology data to make it more useful for physicians, researchers and cancer registries

Check One:

Strongly Agree Agree   Don't Know   Disagree   Strongly Disagree

_____   _____   _____   _____   _____

- As long as the narrative is still part of the record, I would be willing to adapt my procedures for capturing analytic data to include this type of checklist (either in a paper or electronic format).

Check One:

Strongly Agree Agree   Don't Know   Disagree   Strongly Disagree

_____   _____   _____   _____   _____

- Please explain your answers :

- Additional comments:

Appendix M: Ohio RPP Project Assessment Survey
Ohio Department of Health, Ohio Cancer Incidence Surveillance System, RPP Project Assessment
(February, 2005)

Ohio Department of Health, Ohio Cancer Incidence Surveillance System, RPP Project Assessment
February, 2005

Thank you for agreeing to help us evaluate a new way for recording pathology data, a project funded by the Centers for Disease Control and Prevention. All you have to do is to compare the attached pathology reports. In each set, one is formatted like the report now in use at your hospital. The other report for the same specimen has a Summary based on a standardized method for capturing cancer data. These can be developed for all types of cancer, although the examples are all for colorectal cancers. Look these over, then please answer the following:

I believe that the reports containing the College of American Pathologists Tumor Summary are accurate when compared to our current reports.

Y____   N____

If "No," what do you believe is inaccurate?

_____

_____

After looking at a few of these "checklist" reports and comparing them to our standard reports, I like the new ones better with the standardized College of American Pathologists Tumor Summary at the beginning:

Y____   N____

If "Yes," please explain briefly:

_____

_____

I believe that it is important to standardize the way that pathologists record cancer data in order to allow those data to be utilized more fully in terms of using them for research, for reporting to cancer registries, and for cancer surveillance.   Y____   N____

If "No," please comment on your answer

_____

_____

Appendix N: University Hospitals of Cleveland Surgical Pathology Report

UniversityHospitals HealthSystem

UniversityHospitals of Cleveland

Department of Pathology
11100 Euclid Avenue
Cleveland, Ohio 44106-5000
Phone: (216) 844-1817 Fax: (216) 844-1810

SURGICAL PATHOLOGY REPORT

Name: **TEST, CASE**
Accession #: **SS05-1**
Date of Procedure: 4/26/2005
Date Received: 4/26/2005
Date Reported: 4/26/2005

Submitting Physician: DOCTOR XXXX

Med. Rec. #: **02700017**
Date of Visit: **4/8/2003**
Serv/Loc: 042/GENMED
Race: CAUCASIAN
DOB/Sex: 7/5/1967 (Age: 37) M
SS#:
Other External #:
Copy To:

FINAL DIAGNOSIS

See the College of American Pathologists Tumor Summary below.

College of American Pathologists Tumor Summary
A. COLON RESECTION:
--------------- MACROSCOPIC ---------------

Specimen Type:	Right hemicolectomy
	Length of specimen: 100 cm
Tumor Site:	Right (ascending) colon
Tumor Configuration:	Infiltrative
Tumor Size:	Greatest dimension: 25 cm
Intactness of Mesorectum:	Not applicable

--------------- MICROSCOPIC ---------------

Histologic Type:	Adenocarcinoma
Histologic Grade:	Low-grade (well to moderately differentiated)
Pathologic Staging (pTNM):	pT1: Tumor invades submucosa
	pN1: Metastasis in 1 to 3 lymph nodes
	Number of nodes examined: 10
	Number of nodes involved: 1
	pMX: Distant metastasis cannot be assessed
Margins:	Proximal margin involved by invasive carcinoma
	Distal margin uninvolved by invasive carcinoma
	Circumferential (radial) margin - Not applicable
	Mesenteric margin uninvolved by invasive carcinoma
Lymphatic (Small Vessel) Invasion (L):	Absent
Venous (Large Vessel) Invasion (V):	Absent
Perineural Invasion:	Absent
Tumor Border Configuration:	Infiltrating
Tumoral Lymphocytic Response:	Mild to moderate
Additional Pathologic Findings:	None identified

Clinical History:
Colon CA.

Specimens Submitted As:
A: COLON RESECTION

TEST, CASE   Page 1 of 2

Appendix N: University Hospitals of Cleveland Surgical Pathology Report

Glossary: Web Links

1. **ACoS CoC: American College of Surgeons:** http://www.facs.org/
2. **CernerDynamic Healthcare Technologies(Cerner DHT):** http://www.cerner.com/default.asp
3. **C/NET Solutions:** http://www.askcnet.org/
4. **HL7:** http://www.hl7.org/
5. **International Classification of Diseases, Ninth Revision, Clinical Modification (ICD-9-CM):** http://www.cdc.gov/nchs/about/otheract/icd9/abticd9.htm
6. **Logical Observation Identifiers Names and Codes (LOINC):** http://www.regenstrief.org/loinc/
7. **North American Association of Central Cancer Registries, Inc. (NAACCR, Inc.):** http://www.naaccr.org/
8. **National Program of Cancer Registries (NPCR):** http://www.cdc.gov/cancer/npcr/index.htm
9. **Surveillance, Epidemiology, and End Results (SEER):** http://seer.cancer.gov/
10. **SNOMED® International:** http://www.snomed.org/
11. **SNOMED Clinical Terms (SNOMED CT):** http://www.snomed.org/
12. **Statistics Canada:** http://www.statcan.ca/
13. **Public Health Information Network (PHIN):** http://www.cdc.gov/phin/
14. **College of American Pathologists (CAP):** http://www.cap.org/apps/cap.portal
15. **California Cancer Registry:** http://www.ccrcal.org/
16. **Ohio Cancer Registry:** http://www.odh.ohio.gov/odhPrograms/svio/ci_surv/ci_surv1.aspx

Index

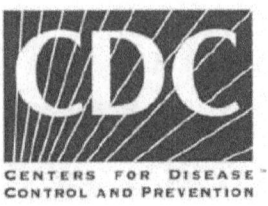

www.ingramcontent.com/pod-product-compliance
Lightning Source LLC
Chambersburg PA
CBHW080300180526
45167CB00006B/2612